EMERGENCY WOUND CARE

Principles and Practice

Donald Demetrios Zukin, MD
Emergency Department
Children's Hospital of Oakland
Oakland, California

Robert Rutha Simon, MD
Department of Emergency Medicine
UCLA-Center for the Health Sciences
Los Angeles, California

Illustrations by **Martha Blake, MA**

AN ASPEN PUBLICATION
Aspen Publishers, Inc.

1987

Rockville, Maryland
Royal Tunbridge Wells

Library of Congress Cataloging-in-Publication Data

Zukin, Donald Demetrios.
Emergency wound care.

"An Aspen publication."
Bibliography: p.
1. Wounds and injuries—Surgery. 2. Surgical
emergencies. I. Simon, Robert R. (Robert Rutha)
II. Title. [DNLM: 1. Emergency Service, Hospital.
2. Wounds and Injuries—therapy. WO 700 Z94e]
RD93.Z85   1987   617'1026   87-14468
ISBN: 0-87189-861-6

The authors have made every effort to ensure the accuracy of the information herein, particularly with regard to drug selection and dose. However, appropriate information sources should be consulted, especially for new or unfamiliar drugs or procedures. It is the responsibility of every practitioner to evaluate the appropriateness of a particular opinion in the context of actual clinical situations and with due consideration to new developments. Authors, editors, and the publisher cannot be held responsible for any typographical or other errors found in this book.

Library of Congress Catalog Card Number: 87-14468
ISBN: 0-87189-861-6

Printed in the United States of America

1   2   3   4   5

Table of Contents

Foreword

In reflecting upon the history of our specialty of emergency medicine, it appears to me that we are guilty of the very sin that we have criticized in other specialties, namely allowing the least-experienced house officers and students to be responsible for tasks that require a significant degree of maturity and clinical expertise and experience. Nowhere is this more true than in the management of wounds.

It is true that in a busy emergency department small soft tissue wounds are not only common, their number can become overwhelming. It is therefore common practice to allow the junior house staff and students to be responsible for wound management. This practice serves many useful purposes. It ensures that the student or junior house officer will be busy for long periods of time, thus preventing one from having to fear what is being done to more complex cases. It ultimately lowers the workload. It even assures patients that their wounds are very serious because it takes so long for their repair. Finally, it amuses the student or house officer because it is fun to sew, and one truly feels like a physician because one is doing something useful.

But there is a serious disadvantage to this practice. Nobody has bothered to instruct the student in how to manage wounds. If there ever had been a suture laboratory, it was given only once a month and the student or house officer

may well have missed it. Attendings are frequently bored with answering the same questions about wounds, so they either avoid the responsibility or write complicated protocols that are placed in computers or handed out, to be thrown away or read and forgotten. Patients may be less than satisfied with a resultant scar that is unnecessarily ugly, and certainly the inexperienced student or house officer does not improve by repeating the same mistakes.

There are many aspects of surgery that cannot be learned from a book. Watching someone experienced, having an opportunity to begin to learn on an easy laceration, and having supervision for the management of complex wounds is ideal. But there is much that can be learned from a book, and building on that pyramid of knowledge, the practical technical tasks are made easier.

Emergency Wound Care is a book that should be mandatory reading for anyone who has responsibility for wound management. For those who have been doing the job for a long time and think they know all about wounds, it will stimulate them into thinking about what their practice actually consists of, and whether they agree or not with the recommended practices, it will be salutary to consider whether positive changes can be integrated into their practices. For the novice, this book represents a beginning of information and practice. There is much here that will be hard to understand without having managed a real wound, but that provides a good reason to own the book and turn to it frequently.

The basics of wound healing are here; no longer will one have to be embarrassed about not even knowing how to start a repair. What needs to be done and, more importantly, why, can be found in this book. Not only are practical details of management addressed, such as what scrub solution to use, and how long to leave sutures in place, but the research physiology of wound repair that has provided the basis for clinical management is also presented.

Because wounds are frequently assigned to the most junior member of the team, they are frequently thought of as trivial problems that are beneath the attention of more experienced physicians. But to approach wounds from this perverted perspective is to miss the excitement of emergency medicine and the fulfillment of much of its clinical practice. Wounds are important to patients: they bleed, they gape, they hurt, and they demand attention. The scar is always there to see, and the incident that produced the wound stays in one's memory in a way matched by few other life events. The way in which physicians interact with wound patients will do much to define not only their personal status, but that of the profession. It is a pleasure to see what good results can be effected with meticulous care and to see the patients' enjoyment of that result.

The faculty member who avoids soft tissue wounds is missing a teaching opportunity unparalleled in emergency medicine. I have had the pleasure of watching many residents, who at the start of their residency carried out wound repair with hesitation, clumsiness, and what can only be accurately defined as motor idiocy, become competent and confident wound repairers. Some of these physicians, I am sad to admit, are now much better than I am. But what price would one pay for having had the opportunity to participate in that evolution?

To any experienced emergency physician who reads this book, I can only hope that you will share the intellectual stimulation that I had with my first reading. There are areas that I don't agree with—not that I have any data with which to refute them other than my own clinical experience; but this is the fun of an autonomous emergency literature. Some of the data, derived from an in-patient surgical literature, I feel sure does not apply to the emergency department. But if the book can excite and challenge my thinking about wound repair after my almost thirty years of experience, I am sure that it will provide information and intellectual stimulation to those just starting on the path of wound repair. My fondest expectation is that it will become the standard text in the field for the obligatory reading of any emergency medicine house officer or student rotating through an emergency department, and that practicing emergency physicians, especially the faculty, will return to this book to challenge, define, and refine their own practices. It might even stimulate some research that will contradict some of the recommendations in the book. Finally, perhaps it will motivate a closer supervision of those wounds that may seem trivial to the pseudosophisticate in the emergency department, but are anything but trivial to the possessor of the wound or a concerned relative.

I will never forget an attending physician who replied to my query about why he didn't let me close the skin of the patient upon whom he was doing a laparotomy: ''That is the only part of my surgery the patient can see.'' If we keep in mind that we will be judged by the resultant scar, the soft tissue wound will assume equal importance to the physician and the patient, which in turn will stimulate us to provide the supervision and care that will effect the best result. The first step in that process is to read and assimilate the material presented so well in the following pages.

Peter Rosen, M.D.

Preface

This text is designed to aid the emergency physician in the treatment of patients with common wounds who present to the emergency department. The book is organized according to the type of injury (i.e., lacerations, burns, abrasions) as well as according to the part of the body that is involved (e.g., regional care). Both basic procedures, such as the simple skin suture, and advanced techniques, such as advancement flaps, are covered.

With the development of emergency medicine as a specialty, there has been an increase in the amount of information about the effects of various therapies, such as wound irrigation and antisepsis. Many classic teachings have been reexamined.

For example, the classic teaching that antiseptic solutions should not be used to prepare the subcutaneous tissues of a wound (''Never put anything into a wound that you would not put into your own eye'') has turned out to be false. Povidone-iodine solution (1 percent) lowers the wound infection rate without causing any necrosis to the subcutaneous tissue (see Chapter 4).

The classic teaching, ''Never close a laceration caused by an animal bite'' is refuted by the fact that there is only a minimal difference in the infection rates between sutured and nonsutured dog bites (see Chapter 9).

Finally, the familiar recommendation to keep the sutured laceration ''clean and dry'' may need to be updated to ''Keep the wound clean and moist.'' In experimental animals, keeping the wound surface moist with the use of occlusive dressings causes a significant increase in the rate of reepithelialization (see Chapter 11).

The bulk of the text, however, deals with the practical aspects of the treatment of burns, abrasions, foreign bodies, and lacerations. The chapters on basic and advanced techniques in suturing and laceration care are designed for students and house officers rotating through the emergency department. The chapters on special techniques and regional care contain reference material that we hope will be suitable for advanced emergency medicine residents and for practicing emergency physicians.

Acknowledgments

We wish to thank our friends and families who provided invaluable help and support for this effort.

We also wish to thank Dr. Peter Rosen of the Denver General Hospital, whose wisdom and experience brought many of the controversial areas of wound care into perspective.

Chapter 1

Wound Healing

SKIN ANATOMY

The skin is composed of two layers, the epidermis above and the dermis below (Fig. 1-1).

The epidermis protects the underlying dermis from infection and dessication. Without the epidermis, cells in the dermis that are exposed to the air dessicate and die.

The epidermis consists of several layers. The basal layer (stratum malpighii) comes into contact with the underlying dermis. The next layer, the stratum granulosum, consists of keratin-containing cells. These cells flatten out and lose their nuclei, forming the top layer, the stratum corneum. The protective stratum corneum hypertrophies greatly in regions of extensive use, such as the palms of the hands and the soles of the feet.

The dermis is high in collagen and accounts for most of the tensile strength of the skin. The dermis consists of an upper, papillary layer that interdigitates into the epidermis, and a lower, reticular layer that is made up of dense connective tissue. The nutrient vessels of the skin arborize into dermal capillaries.

Below the dermis is a layer of loose connective and adipose tissue called the *hypodermis*, or more commonly, the subcutaneous fat. The thickness of this layer varies greatly in different regions of the body. In the abdomen, thigh, and buttocks, for example, the adipose tissue is quite thick, while beneath the skin of the upper eyelids

it is nonexistent. The large vessels and nerves of the skin travel within this layer.

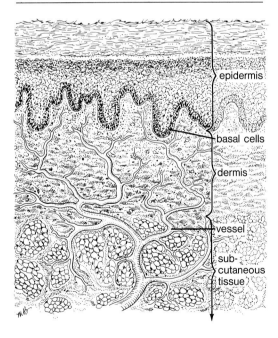

Figure 1-1 The anatomy of the skin. The top layer, the epidermis, consists of epithelial cells, and serves to protect the deep tissue from desiccation and infection. The middle layer, the dermis, contains fibroblasts which produce the collagen that gives the skin its tensile strength. The blood vessels of the skin are contained within the dermis. (This illustration is not to scale: the dermis is in reality many times the thickness of the epidermis.)

SKIN INJURIES

Lacerations

General

A *laceration* is simply a cut through the skin. If only the epidermis is involved, there will be no bleeding. However, lacerations that are deep enough to involve dermal capillaries will bleed. Because the dermal papillae intercalate into the epidermis at various depths, superficial lacerations frequently demonstrate small, punctate regions of bleeding where dermal vessels have been severed. By contrast, deeper lacerations involve the dermis along the whole extent of the injury, and the bleeding is more uniform. If only the upper part of the dermis is involved, gaping of the wound is minimal, because the deep fibrous reticular layer keeps the edges apposed. However, if the laceration reaches the layer of subcutaneous fat, the wound edges will tend to gape open.

Classification of Lacerations

Shear Lacerations. Shear lacerations are those caused by sharp objects, such as knife blades and glass shards. There is little damage to the tissues adjacent to the wound. Shear lacerations heal rapidly and with minimal scarring because of the health of the tissues at the wound edges.

Tension Lacerations. Unlike the shear laceration, which is caused by an object cutting the skin, in *tension lacerations* the skin strikes a flat surface and, in essence, rips because of the tissue stresses caused by the impact. There is no bone directly below the region of skin that is struck. An example of a tension injury is the slightly ragged linear laceration on the palm that occurs when a patient falls down on a hard surface and breaks the fall with his or her hands. Because there is contusion of the neighboring soft tissues, tension lacerations heal with more scarring than shear lacerations.

Compression Lacerations. Compression lacerations occur when the tissue is caught between a bone and an external hard surface. The result is that the skin bursts, often causing a stellate pattern to appear. Compression lacerations frequently result from a fall in which the forehead hits the pavement.

Because there is a marked degree of injury to the skin adjacent to the laceration itself, compression injuries heal the most poorly, and with the greatest degree of scarring.

Combination Lacerations. Combination lacerations have characteristics of both shear and compression injuries. An example is an injury that occurs when a dull edge, such as the corner of a table strikes a bony prominence. The resulting laceration is linear, as with a shear injury, but the wound edges are crushed, as with a compression injury.

Abrasions

An *abrasion* is an injury in which various layers of skin are scraped away. With superficial abrasions only the cornified epidermis is lost. There is no bleeding, although there may be exudation of fluid. Deeper abrasions reach the dermal papillae, and consequently there is hemorrhaging. Full-thickness abrasions remove both the epidermis and the dermis, leaving the subcutaneous fat cells exposed to the air.

Burns

First-Degree Burn

In a *first-degree burn*, the epidermis is injured, but the dermis remains intact. The skin displays erythema, but no blister formation. Several days following the injury the skin may peel.

Second-Degree Burn (Partial Thickness)

In a *second-degree burn,* the injury is more extensive, with some dermal necrosis and blistering of the skin. The dermal vessels and nerves, however, survive. Consequently perfusion and sensation remain intact. The epidermal cells within the hair follicles and skin appendages also survive.

With deep second-degree burns the deep dermal vessels, which are initially patent, can leak fluid, leading to sludging and eventually thrombosis. Thus over a period of 1 to 3 days a partial-thickness injury may convert into a full-thickness injury. In laboratory studies, burned tissue (epidermis and upper dermis) which is excised and then transplanted to a healthy, noninjured vascular bed will have greater chances of survival than burned tissue left in the original site.[105]

Any insult to the burned region, such as a secondary infection, makes the conversion of a partial-thickness burn into a full-thickness burn more likely, while the immediate application of cold water to the burned area can keep the thermal injury from reaching the deep vessels and prevent the burn from becoming full thickness.

Third-Degree Burn (Full Thickness)

In a *third-degree burn*, both the epidermis and the dermis necrose. There is thrombosis of the blood vessels. The skin appears leathery and lacks both sensation and capillary refill.

Fourth-Degree Burn

In a *fourth-degree burn* there is full-thickness skin necrosis with accompanying damage to underlying muscle, bone, and tendon (as occurs with electrical burns).

NORMAL HEALING

Basic Healing[103,190]

The skin has a basic pattern of healing for all injuries that are deep enough to involve the dermis. Without the protective cover of the epidermis, the superficial cells in the dermis desiccate and die. Combined with serous fluid from the wound, these necrotic cells form the familiar wound eschar.

Healing occurs from the edges of the wound and from intact hair follicles, sweat glands, and sebaceous glands. A rapid infiltration of inflammatory cells occurs in the first two days. The early infiltrate consists of polymorphonuclear leukocytes and macrophages, but later the infiltrate consists primarily of macrophages. By the third day fibroblasts appear, which lay down a gelatinous matrix which later turns into collagen. Into this matrix new capillaries bud from existing blood vessels at the periphery of the wound. The arborization of new vessels, termed *neovascularization*, can lend a violaceous hue to the periphery of the wound which at times can look like early cellulitis.

Over the advancing lattice of monocytes, fibroblasts, and budding capillaries migrate the epithelial cells of the regenerating epidermis. These epithelial cells will not migrate over the necrotic fibroblasts of the eschar, but cleave beneath the eschar to the new, healthy dermis being created.

The healing rim of fibroblasts, inflammatory cells, capillary buds, and new epidermal cells is familiar to the physician as granulation tissue. When the new tissue completely closes the defect left by the wound, the capillary buds from each side anastomose, and the overlying epidermal layer fuses from both sides. As the basal epidermal cells differentiate to form the cornified layer, the eschar peels away. If the eschar is removed prematurely, the nascent epithelial cells are peeled away as well.

The speed with which the wound closes is not solely dependent on the speed of migration of the epithelial cells. In addition, the new fibrous tissue at the wound perimeter contains contractile cells, called *myofibroblasts*, which cause the diameter of the wound to decrease in size over time. This process is termed *wound contraction*.

With time the collagen fibers within the scar remodel, forming bundles which are more compact and stronger than the immature fibers. As a result the tensile strength of the scar continues to increase for several months, reaching a maximum 6 to 8 months following the injury.

Although the fully healed wound consists of a layer of epidermis atop a layer of dermis, the appearance is often not that of normal skin. Especially with deep wounds, the regenerated tissue lacks the dermal papillae which are normally interspersed throughout the epidermis. Therefore the resultant scar often appears flat and shiny.

Healing by Wound Type

Abrasions

If only the top of the epidermis is abraded away, then healing will be by direct regeneration from the underlying basal cells. If the entire epidermal layer is lost, then epidermal cells from hair follicles and skin appendages within the dermis multiply and migrate out over the dermis to form the new epidermal layer. If the injury is so extensive as to remove both the epidermis and the dermis (with the hair follicles and skin glands), then healing takes place entirely from granulation tissue at the edges of the wound.

Lacerations

In lacerations that are closed with sutures or skin tape, a small eschar of dried serous fluid and desiccated dermal cells forms on top of the wound. Beneath this eschar epidermal cells migrate out from both wound edges, meeting in the midline beneath the eschar.

Below the new epidermal layer, new capillary bridges form, while fibroblasts proliferate and lay down new collagen to repair the dermal defect.

In lacerations that are left open the pattern of healing is essentially the same, except that the size of the eschar is multiplied many times. The metabolic demands to repair the larger defects are much greater than those to repair smaller defects of lacerations that have been closed primarily. Hence patients with marginal perfusion (as in diabetes or peripheral vascular disease) will often be unable to heal a laceration that is left open, but are able to heal one that is sutured closed.[104] Chapter 5, Basic Laceration Repair, addresses laceration repair by primary, secondary, and tertiary intent.

Burns[105]

First-degree burns heal by regeneration of the injured epidermal cells from underlying basal cells, as occurs with superficial abrasions.

In second-degree burns the epidermis is regenerated from the neighboring intact epidermis, and from epidermal cells found in hair follicles and sweat and sebaceous glands. If the burn blister remains intact there is no eschar and no necrosis of the superficial cells of the dermis. The epidermal cells are therefore able to migrate relatively rapidly over the intact dermis to form the new epidermal layer. If the blister breaks, the superficial dermis will necrose and become incorporated into the eschar. Healing is then delayed by approximately 25 percent because the regenerating epidermal cells must burrow beneath an eschar.

Third-degree burns heal by the formation of granulation tissue at the periphery of the burn. The leathery eschar separates from the underlying tissue after a period of 1 to several weeks.

ABNORMAL HEALING

Keloid Scars[106]

A *keloid scar* is a large, thick scar that hypertrophies to the extent that it actually exceeds the size of the original wound. Keloids occur more frequently in individuals with deeply pigmented skin, in pregnant women, and in adolescents. In normal scar maturation, simultaneous collagen formation and collagenolysis occur. The basic defect in keloid formation is that collagen formation exceeds collagen breakdown. The association with pigmentation has led to speculation that melanocyte stimulating hormone may be involved in keloid scar formation.

Hypertrophic Scars

Like a keloid scar, a hypertrophic scar is abnormally thick. And, as with a keloid scar, collagen formation exceeds collagen breakdown. Unlike keloid scars, however, hypertrophic scars do not extend beyond the limits of the original injury. In addition, hypertrophic scars are more likely to involute with time.

Hypertrophic scars are especially likely to form in areas of motion, such as over joints. Thus hypertrophic scars frequently occur over the knees and shoulders. In addition, hypertrophic scars commonly occur following wounds over the sternum.

FACTORS AFFECTING HEALING

Oxygen[145]

The local oxygen tension in the wound cavity drops off rapidly with increasing distance from the intact skin edge. Even when supplemental oxygen is provided to the patient, the oxygen tension a few millimeters from the wound edge rapidly falls toward zero.[104]

Interestingly, the low oxygen tension at the wound edge appears to be a stimulus for wound repair. When the oxygen tension falls below 10 torr, angiogenesis and cell migration are activated. Fibroblasts synthesize collagen at the maximum rate when the oxygen tension is between 15 and 30 torr. Proliferation of tissue cells at the wound edge is at a maximum when the oxygen tension is between 15 and 30 torr. However, oxygen tensions above 30 torr are necessary for the body's defenses against bacterial invasion to be at a maximum.

Nutrition

Nutritional deficiencies adversely affect wound healing. Protein and carbohydrates are needed to provide the energy and the basic building blocks for repair. Vitamin A aids in the formation of a new epithelial layer and the formation of healthy collagen. Vitamin C is also necessary for the formation of normal collagen because it aids in the formation of covalent bonds between the collagen fibers. Deficiencies of iron and zinc impair the healing process.

Although adequate nutrition enhances healing, overenthusiastic supplementation of certain nutrients can be harmful. For example, zinc in excess decreases both cell chemotaxis and bacterial phagocytosis.[145] Similarly, excess vitamin E diminishes wound tensile strength in experimental animals.[145]

Foreign Bodies

As mentioned above, tissue hypoxia stimulates the formation of new capillaries, and the migration and proliferation of fibroblasts and other cells. Normally, as healing proceeds, the oxygen tension gradually rises and these processes then recede.

The oxygen tension around a foreign body remains near zero, even as healing proceeds. This persistently low tension causes angiogenesis and cell proliferation to continue for an abnormally long period of time, delaying the formation of the mature scar.

Also, a foreign body may serve as a nidus for infection, and once the infection occurs, the low oxygen tension adjacent to the foreign body impairs the bacteriocidal activity of polymorphonuclear leukocytes.

Medications[104,145]

Several systemic medications adversely affect wound healing. Corticosteroids inhibit formation of the epithelial layer and also decrease normal scar contraction. Antineoplastic drugs interfere with cell division. Anticoagulants impair hemostasis.

Some medications appear to aid in healing. The antiprostaglandin agent ibuprofen appears to decrease microvascular occlusion, and to increase cellular immunity in burn victims.[145] In some studies phenytoin appears to increase wound tensile strength by inhibiting collagen breakdown.[145]

Occlusive Dressings

Occlusive wound dressings, such as polyurethane film (Op-site), by keeping the wound surface hydrated, prevent the dessication and subsequent necrosis of the exposed dermis. The typical eschar hence does not form. As a consequence, epithelialization is dramatically accelerated, since the migrating cells no longer need to cleave away the overlying eschar (see Chapter 11).

Chapter 2

Materials

INSTRUMENTS

Only a few basic instruments are required for the repair of most wounds. These include a needle holder, forceps, a no. 15 scalpel, and scissors.

Needle Holders

Needle holders are constructed with jaws that are both shorter and thicker than in standard clamps. The strong jaws can securely grasp a needle without bending.

Long needle holders, useful in dealing with deep abdominal wounds, are rarely required in emergency department wound repair.

Needle holders are available with either smooth or ridged (corrugated) grasping surfaces, as shown in Figure 2-1. The smooth surface, on the one hand, is better able to grasp fine suture material, such as 6-0 nylon. Fine materials tend to pull through the ridges of the corrugated surface. The ridged surface, on the other hand, holds large needles more securely, and thus is useful in repairing scalp lacerations, for example.

Clamps

Clamps are sometimes needed to grasp small vessels in order to ligate them. Since most simple lacerations do not require ligation of vessels,

usually a single straight clamp will suffice. Additional clamps can be sterilized individually for use as the need arises. For example, two clamps are required to divide a vessel in the middle of a wound.

Forceps

Forceps are available in various sizes, and with either smooth or toothed grasping surfaces.

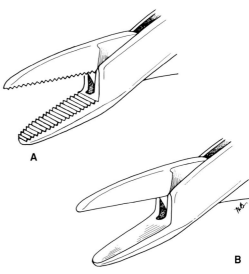

Figure 2-1. Needle holder blades with ridged (**A**) and smooth (**B**) surfaces.

Although the smooth surface would appear to be less traumatic than the toothed surface, this is generally not true. Because tissue tends to slip more easily from smooth-surfaced forceps, there is a greater tendency to crush the tissues than when using toothed forceps. Either type, however, is adequate, as long as the physician treats the tissues as gently as possible.

Skin Hooks

Skin hooks allow for manipulation of the wound edge without crushing tissue. If a standard skin hook is not available, such a hook can easily be constructed by inserting the end of a cotton-tipped applicator into the hub of a 22-gauge needle, and then bending the tip of the needle into an arc with a needle holder (Fig. 2-2).

Scissors

A small, sharp iris scissors is the most useful type for wound repair. Iris scissors can be used

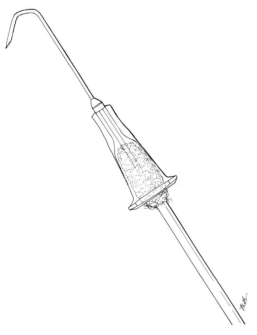

Figure 2-2. A skin hook can be constructed by inserting a cotton-tipped applicator into the hub of a 22-gauge needle, and then bending the tip of the needle.

for trimming tissue edges and cutting sutures. Larger scissors are useful for cutting bandages during dressing changes.

Retractors

A set of small retractors can be invaluable in exploring a wound in a vital area, such as the hand or the wrist, to see if there is damage to a nerve, artery, tendon, or joint capsule. Large retractors are usually not required for emergency department wound repair.

NEEDLES

Needles are either straight (for use with the hands) or curved (for use with needle holders). The most commonly used curved needle is the ⅜ circle.

There are two basic types of needles: the tapered needle, which has a circular cross-sectional configuration, and the cutting needle, which has a triangular cross-sectional configuration. In the standard cutting needle the cutting surface (apex of the triangle) is on the inner aspect of the curve. In the reverse cutting needle the cutting surface (apex of the triangle) is on the outer surface of the curve (Fig. 2-3). Many manufacturers label both the cutting and the reverse cutting needle simply as a "cutting needle."

A tapered needle leaves a smaller hole, but cutting needles are better able to pass through tough skin.

There are two grades of needles, cuticular and plastic. Plastic needles are honed more sharply than cuticular needles, and are thus more expensive. Plastic needles are usually designated by a P (plastic) or PS (plastic surgery). Cuticular needles are usually designated C (cuticular) or FS (for skin). The number following the letter indicates the size of the needle. With most brands, the larger the number, the smaller the needle.

The needles most commonly used in emergency departments come attached (swaged) to the suture. Using these needles creates less trauma because there is no enlarged eye of the needle to pass through the tissue.

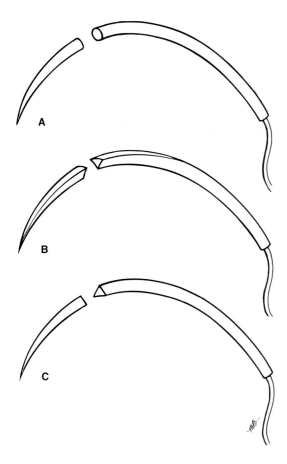

Figure 2-3. Needle configurations. The tapered needle has a circular cross-section (**A**). The cutting needle has a triangular cross-section, with the cutting surface on the inner aspect of the curve of the needle (**B**). The reverse cutting needle also has a triangular cross-section, but the cutting surface is found on the outer aspect of the curve of the needle (**C**).

Small needles are used for finer repairs, for example, when treating facial lacerations. Larger needles are useful for taking bigger bites of tissue, such as when repairing scalp lacerations.

SUTURE MATERIALS[1,3,50,54,55,106,123,150,164,176]

Nonabsorbable Sutures

Silk

Silk was one of the first nonabsorbable sutures. Silk has several desirable qualities. It lays flat when tied (unlike many synthetic materials), and is therefore easier to handle. Silk, when braided, forms a secure knot.

Although easy to handle, silk is not the ideal suture material for routine emergency department use. Being a foreign protein, silk engenders a host tissue reaction. Silk sutures have a much higher infection potential than synthetic monofilament sutures such as nylon or polypropylene. In one animal experiment, although 10^6 bacteria were required to produce a wound infection in a standard-sized wound, only 10^2 bacteria were needed to cause an infection when silk sutures were present in the wound.[55] Human experiments in this area are lacking, however. The infection potentiating aspects of silk limit its use to uncontaminated wounds in well-perfused areas of the body, such as the face. Silk is useful for repair of lacerations of the nipple, lip, and nose, where stiffer suture materials are uncomfortable to the patient.

Cotton

Cotton possesses many of the qualities of silk. Cotton sutures lie flat and hold knots well, but also have the undesirable attributes of high infection potential and moderate tissue reactivity.[50]

Nylon and Polypropylene

Nylon (Ethylon) and polypropylene (Prolene) are synthetic materials which have significantly lower infection potentials and tissue reactivities than cotton or silk. This low infection potential makes them the sutures of choice for skin closure of most lacerations treated in the emergency department. However, unlike silk and cotton, these materials do not tend to lie flat during suturing, hence they are more difficult to use. Also, the lack of braiding decreases the security of knots tied with these materials. Therefore both nylon and polypropylene sutures need to be tied with four to five "throws" per knot.

Dacron

In experimental wounds, Dacron sutures have an infection potential that is greater than nylon or polypropylene but less than silk or cotton.[50]

Dacron sutures are easier to work with and hold knots better than nylon and polypropylene.

Metal Sutures

Metal sutures offer many of the advantages of nylon and polypropylene, including low tissue reactivity and low infection potential. However, metal is very difficult to use and highly irritating to the patient.

Absorbable Suture Materials

Plain Cat Gut

Gut is the classic absorbable suture material. The mechanism of absorption is primarily phagocytosis by macrophages. Plain gut sutures continue to hold tensile strength for approximately 7 days. Gut has the disadvantage of high tissue reactivity and increased pyogenicity, compared to synthetic absorbable materials such as polyglycolic acid (PGA).[50]

Chromic Cat Gut

Plain gut can be treated with chromium ion solution to yield a suture which retains its tensile strength for approximately 2 to 3 weeks. Like plain gut, it also has the disadvantages of high pyogenicity and tissue reactivity.

Synthetic Absorbable Sutures

The synthetic absorbable sutures PGA (Dexon) and polyglactin 910 (Vycril) cause less tissue reactivity and have lower pyogenicity than plain or chromic gut.[50] These materials are absorbed by enzymatic hydrolysis, rather than by monophage phagocytosis. PGA and polyglactin 910 retain tensile strength for 60 days or more, thus providing prolonged support to a healing wound.

However, these synthetic materials also have drawbacks. They do not glide through tissues as well as plain or chromic gut. Snags tend to occur, which makes knot tying more tedious.

SKIN TAPES[54,150]

Skin tapes (Steri-Strips, Clearon, and Shur-strips) can be used in place of sutures to repair surface lacerations. In animal studies, contaminated wounds closed with skin tape have a significantly lower incidence of infection than those closed with conventional sutures.[54] Skin tapes also offer the advantage of not causing suture marks, and of not requiring a return visit for removal.

Tapes, however, are not practical in areas of motion or in areas that will become wet.

The sticking power of tapes is enhanced by pretreating the skin adjacent to the wound with an adhesive agent, such as tincture of benzoin.

Chapter 3

Anesthesia

ANESTHETIC AGENTS

There are two main classes of local anesthetics, the esters and the amides (Table 3-1). If a patient has demonstrated an allergic reaction to an agent within a group, then he or she should be considered allergic to all agents in that group, but not necessarily to agents in the other group. For example, a patient who develops hives when administered lidocaine should not be treated subsequently with any amide anesthetic agent, but may be treated with an ester agent, such as procaine.

The esters include such agents as Novocain and procaine. These agents produce a slightly higher incidence of allergic reactions than the amides. Also, the esters tend to have a slower onset of action. Due to these limitations, the esters are usually reserved for patients who are allergic to amides.

The amides include agents such as lidocaine and bupivacaine. As mentioned above, the onset of action tends to be faster than with the esters, and the incidence of allergic reactions less.

Table 3-1 lists the properties of various agents.

The addition of epinephrine to local anesthetic solutions both prolongs the duration of action and increases the total permissible subcutaneous dose a patient can receive. Thus the dose of plain lidocaine should not exceed 4 mg/kg, or in an average adult about 28 cc of a 1 percent solution (280 mg). By contrast, one can give 7 mg/kg of lidocaine with epinephrine for infiltration, which in an average adult equals 49 cc of a 1 percent solution (490 mg). *Epinephrine should only be used in regions with good perfusion (such as the scalp, cheek, and forehead), and never in the fingers, toes, penis, apex of the nose, or any other regions fed by single arteries, because ischemic necrosis can result.* Epinephrine increases the rate of wound infection in experimental animals, and hence whenever possible its use should be reserved for clean lacerations.[130]

Axiom: Anesthetic solutions with epinephrine should not be used in the fingers, toes, penis, or apex of the nose.

ANESTHETIC TECHNIQUES

Topical Anesthetic

Certain anesthetic agents can provide fair anesthesia when applied topically to the area one wishes to numb. Cocaine, tetracaine, americaine, and lidocaine are the agents most commonly used as topical agents. TAC, a combination of tetracaine, adrenalin, and cocaine is commonly used in treating small wounds in young children.

Table 3-1 Local Anesthetics[196]

		Amides
Agent	Duration	Maximum Adult Dose (mg)
Bupivacaine (= Marcaine)	4–8 hr	175 (plain) 250 (with epinephrine)
Etidocaine	4–8 hr	200 (plain) 300 (with epinephrine)
Lidocaine (= Xylocaine)	30–120 min	300 (plain) 500 (with epinephrine)
Mepivacaine (= Carbocaine)	90–180 min	300 (plain) 400 (with epinephrine)
		Esters
Tetracaine (= Pontocaine)	Long acting	100 (approximately)
Benzocaine (topical only)	Short acting	Not known
Chloroprocaine (= Nesacaine)	Short acting	600 (plain) 750 (with epinephrine)
Cocaine (topical only)	Medium	200 (= 5 ml of 4%) (some report toxic reactions with lower doses)
Procaine (= Novocain)	30–45 min	500 (plain) 600 (with epinephrine)

TAC solution can be prepared by mixing the ingredients to the following concentrations: tetracaine 0.5 percent, epinephrine 1:2,000, and cocaine 4 percent. The total dose used should not exceed 5 cc in adults. The safe dose for use in children is not known.

The topical anesthetic agent first is poured onto a sterile gauze, and then the gauze is held directly over the wound. The gauze is held in place for approximately 10 minutes.

In clinical studies of TAC, the topical anesthetic provided adequate numbness in about two-thirds of patients.[189] *Caution:* The total safe dose of anesthetic for any patient should never be exceeded, even when applying the agent topically. Cocaine overdosages have occurred following the use of TAC in young children. Even though the agents are applied topically, systemic absorption will occur. Because of the potential for systemic toxicity, the authors do not recommend the routine use of TAC in the emergency department setting.

Cryo-Anesthesia

Partial local anesthesia can be obtained by holding a moistened ice cube on the skin for approximately 5 minutes. Alternatively, commercial coolant solutions are available which can be sprayed onto the skin surface. Both techniques offer only temporary anesthesia, but are useful prior to injecting the skin with anesthetic, particularly in pediatric patients.

Local Infiltration

Subcutaneous Infiltration

Local infiltration into the dermis is probably the most common technique of local anesthesia. For lacerations, enter directly into the dermis through the open wound edge, as this is much less painful for the patient, and there is no evidence that this technique increases the rate of wound infection (Fig. 3-1).

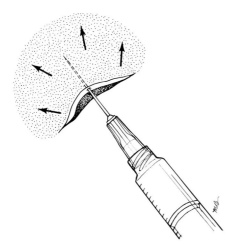

Figure 3-1 Local infiltration. Note that the anesthetic is injected via the wound edge, which causes less pain than injecting through intact skin.

Aspirate back prior to injecting the solution, to be sure that the needle is not in a vessel. Remember, the maximum safe dosages are for subcutaneous, not intravenous administration.

The more slowly the agent is administered, the less discomfort there is for the patient. Using a narrow-caliber needle, such as 25 or 27 gauge, causes less pain to the patient. One should instill the agent beneath the skin surface, raising a wheal in the region to be anesthetized. If the anesthetic is placed too deeply (i.e., in the adipose layer), adequate anesthesia will not be obtained.

Intradermal Infiltration

Interestingly, injection of *any* solution, including saline, intradermally (as in the technique used to give PPD skin tests) yields transient but full anesthesia in the area infiltrated. The increased fluid pressure in the top layer of the skin seems to inactivate the skin's sensory organs. This method, however, is of limited usefulness because only a small area can be anesthetized.

Field Block

In the field block technique, the anesthetic solution is infiltrated beneath the skin in a dia-

mond shape around the wound, as shown in Figure 3-2. As in local infiltration, aspirate back before injecting the solution.

The field block has the advantage of not disrupting the architecture of the wound. This preservation of the normal architecture can be of great advantage, particularly about the face, where malalignment of even 1 mm can worsen the cosmetic appearance of the repair. The main disadvantage of the field block technique is that more anesthetic must be injected than with local infiltration.

Regional Block

In a regional block, one anesthetizes the sensory nerves serving the region to be anesthetized. The regional block technique preserves the architecture of the region to be repaired, and

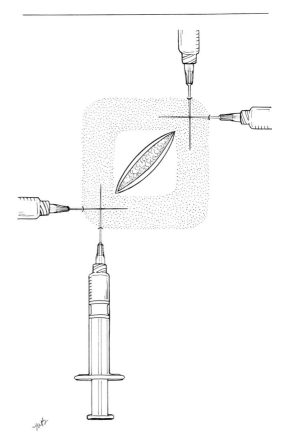

Figure 3-2 Field block. A diamond-shaped pattern is made around the wound. This technique offers the advantage of not distorting the skin edges of the laceration itself.

usually requires a lower total dose of anesthetic solution than used for a field block. The regional block is especially useful for an area that is innervated by only one to two sensory nerves, such as the finger. The technique is not as useful in an area such as the scalp, which is supplied by several sensory nerves.

The anesthetic is placed just adjacent to the appropriate nerve. Ideally, the location of the nerve is first confirmed by inducing paresthesia with the needle. Then the needletip is pulled back 1 to 2 mm from the nerve, and the anesthetic solution is injected at that location. The physician should avoid infiltrating the anesthetic directly into the nerve bundle itself, to minimize the risk of causing nerve damage. In actual practice the incidence of permanent peripheral nerve dysfunction after regional block fortunately is low. As always, aspirate back before injecting, to be certain the needle is not in an artery or vein.

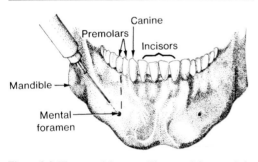

Figure 3-3 The mental foramen. The mental foramen is in the anterior mandible, just below the second premolar. *Source:* Reprinted from *Procedures and Techniques in Emergency Medicine* (p 88) by RR Simon and BE Brenner with permission of the Williams & Wilkins Company, Baltimore, © 1982.

SELECTED NERVE BLOCKS OF THE FACE

Mental Nerve Block

Sensory Distribution

The mental nerve exists just below the second lower premolar and innervates both the skin and mucosa of the ipsilateral lower lip, as shown in Figures 3-3 and 3-4. The nerve does not supply the lower part of the chin, and hence is more useful for lip than for chin lacerations. Performing bilateral mental nerve blocks provides anesthesia to the entire lower lip. Following a mental nerve block, the patient must be cautioned against eating until sensation has returned. Otherwise, he or she may inadvertently chew on the numb lip.

Technique

There are two methods for performing the mental nerve block. In the first, the skin overlying the foramen is prepped with alcohol, and then the needle enters the skin directly over the foramen. The second method is the intraoral approach. First the mucosa in the sulcus of the lower lip is sprayed with topical lidocaine. Then the needle enters this sulcus somewhat anterior to the second premolar, as shown in Figure 3-5. In the authors' experience the intraoral approach is less painful for the patient.

For both techniques, inject about 1 cc of anesthetic solution directly over the region of the foramen, and an additional ¾ cc to the left and

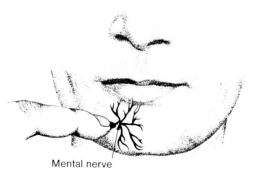

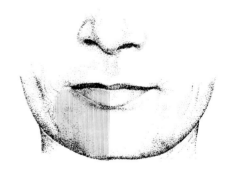

Figure 3-4 The mental nerve supplies sensation to the skin and mucosa of the lower lip. *Source:* Reprinted from *Procedures and Techniques in Emergency Medicine* (p 88) by RR Simon and BE Brenner with permission of the Williams & Wilkins Company, Baltimore, © 1982.

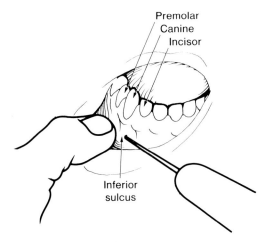

Figure 3-5 Intraoral approach—mental nerve block. The needle enters the mucosa of the inferior sulcus, and then is directed inferiorly and posteriorly to the mental foramen. *Source:* Reprinted from *Procedures and Techniques in Emergency Medicine* (p 88) by RR Simon and BE Brenner with permission of the Williams & Wilkins Company, Baltimore, © 1982.

right of the foramen. Injecting anesthetic solution with epinephrine will prolong the duration of the block.

Infraorbital Nerve Block

Anatomy

The infraorbital nerve exits from the infraorbital foramen which is located slightly medial to the mid-portion of the infraorbital ridge (Fig. 3-6). This nerve provides sensation to the upper lip, as well as to part of the nose and face, as shown in Figure 3-7.

Technique

The foramen can usually be palpated beneath the orbital ridge. The foramen can be approached either directly, from the overlying skin, as indicated by the needle in Figure 3-6A, or by an intraoral approach. For the intraoral approach, enter the superior gingival sulcus just medial to the canine tooth on the side to be blocked. Then advance the needle toward the ipsilateral foramen, using the index finger of the hand not holding the syringe to guide the needle. For both approaches inject about 1 cc of anesthetic at the estimated location of the foramen, and an additional ¾ cc to either side.

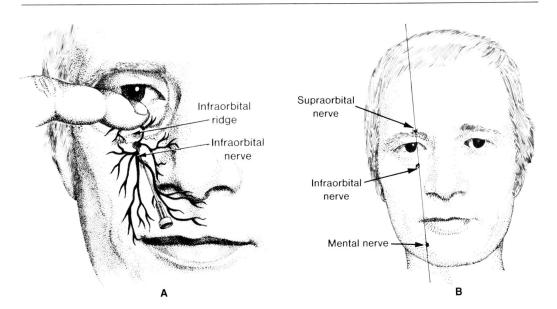

Figure 3-6 The infraorbital nerve. The infraorbital foramen is located inferior to the infraorbital ridge, just medial to the midline (**A**). The infraorbital foramen forms a line with the supraorbital and the mental foramina (**B**). This relationship is useful to use in patients in whom it is difficult to palpate the infraorbital foramen due to swelling of the cheek. *Source:* Reprinted from *Procedures and Techniques in Emergency Medicine* (p 92) by RR Simon and BE Brenner with permission of the Williams & Wilkins Company, Baltimore, © 1982.

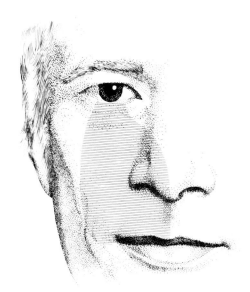

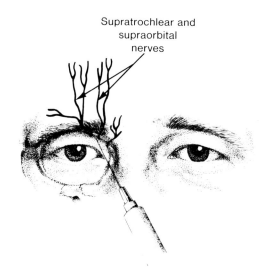
Supratrochlear and supraorbital nerves

Figure 3-7 Sensory distribution of the infraorbital nerve. *Source:* Reprinted from *Procedures and Techniques in Emergency Medicine* (p 92) by RR Simon and BE Brenner with permission of the Williams & Wilkins Company, Baltimore, © 1982.

Figure 3-8 Supraorbital (lateral) and supratrochlear nerves. The nerves exit from foramina located along the medial aspect of the superior orbital ridge. *Source:* Reprinted from *Procedures and Techniques in Emergency Medicine* (p 90) by RR Simon and BE Brenner with permission of the Williams & Wilkins Company, Baltimore, © 1982.

The intraoral approach is slightly harder to master, but is usually more comfortable for the patient.

Caution: With both techniques be sure to stay inferior to the inferior orbital ridge, or else there is a real risk of injecting into the orbit or even the globe. If the technique is used on a child, be sure the child is well immobilized before proceeding.

Supraorbital and Supratrochlear Nerve Blocks

Anatomy

The supraorbital and supratrochlear nerves exit from their respective foramina along the medial border of the superior orbital ridge, as shown in Figure 3-8. These nerves provide sensation to the forehead and anterior scalp. Figure 3-9 demonstrates the distribution of anesthesia from bilateral blocks of these nerves.

Technique

The supraorbital foramen is usually easy to palpate. After the foramen is located inject 1 cc over the foramen, and an additional ¾ cc lateral

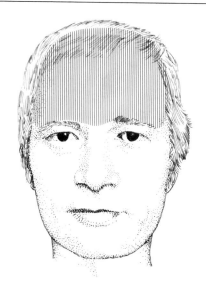

Figure 3-9 The shaded area indicates the pattern of anesthesia from bilateral supraorbital and supratrochlear nerve blocks. *Source:* Reprinted from *Procedures and Techniques in Emergency Medicine* (p 90) by RR Simon and BE Brenner with permission of the Williams & Wilkins Company, Baltimore, © 1982.

to the foramen. Then, without removing the needle, reposition the needle to the estimated location of the supratrochlear nerve (i.e., about

½ to 1 cm medial to where the supraorbital foramen was palpated), and inject an additional 1 cc of anesthetic, as shown in Figure 3-10.

It is easiest to perform the block if one first pulls up on the ipsilateral brow and injects through the thin skin of the upper lid. *Caution:* Always stay at or superior to the level of the superior orbital ridge, otherwise the needle might enter the orbit or even the globe itself. When performing the technique on a child, be sure the child is immobilized (and possibly sedated) before proceeding.

An alternative technique for anesthetizing the forehead is to lay a wheal along the forehead just above the brows, as shown in Figure 3-11.

SELECTED REGIONAL NERVE BLOCKS OF THE UPPER EXTREMITY

Median Nerve Block

Anatomy

At the proximal flexor crease of the wrist, the median nerve courses just ulnar to the flexor carpi radialis, as shown in Figure 3-12.

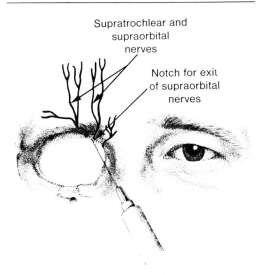

Supratrochlear and supraorbital nerves

Notch for exit of supraorbital nerves

Figure 3-10 Supraorbital and supratrochlear nerve blocks. The nerves pictured indicate where to inject the anesthetic. *Source:* Reprinted from *Procedures and Techniques in Emergency Medicine* (p 91) by RR Simon and BE Brenner with permission of the Williams & Wilkins Company, Baltimore, © 1982.

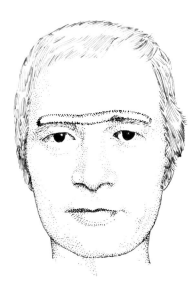

Figure 3-11 An alternative technique to anesthetize the forehead and anterior scalp is to lay a wheal of anesthetic solution just above the eyebrows. *Source:* Reprinted from *Procedures and Techniques in Emergency Medicine* (p 91) by RR Simon and BE Brenner with permission of the Williams & Wilkins Company, Baltimore, © 1982.

The median nerve block anesthetizes the palmar aspect of the thumb, index, and middle fingers, as well as the radial half of the ring finger and the radial half of the palm.

Technique

First locate the flexor carpi radialis by having the patient make a fist and then flex the wrist against resistance. This maneuver also makes the adjacent palmaris longus tendon prominent. In patients without a palmaris longus tendon, the landmark palpable ulnar to the flexor carpi radialis is the flexor digitorum superficialis tendons. Inject immediately adjacent (radially) to the palmaris longus tendon at the level of the proximal flexor crease (Fig. 3-13).

In patients without a palmaris longus tendon, inject radial to the flexor digitorum superficialis tendons.

The median nerve is deep to the flexor retinaculum, therefore one must go through the retinaculum before coming to the nerve. When the needle comes into contact with the nerve, paresthesias will occur in the thumb and first three fingers. Pull back slightly and then instill 2 cc of

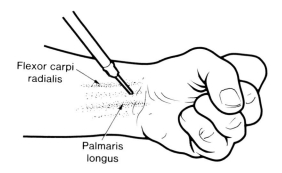

Figure 3-13 The median nerve block. Inject just radial to the palmaris longus tendon at the level of the proximal flexor crease of the wrist. In patients without a palmaris longus tendon, inject radial to the flexor digitorum superficialis tendons. *Source:* Reprinted from *Procedures and Techniques in Emergency Medicine* (p 102) by RR Simon and BE Brenner with permission of the Williams & Wilkins Company, Baltimore, © 1982.

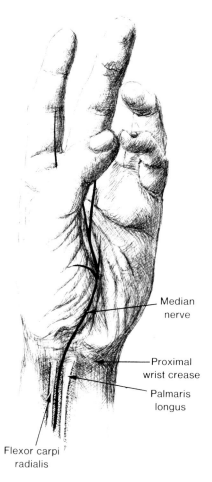

Figure 3-12 The median nerve. At the proximal wrist crease the nerve lies just ulnar to the flexor carpi radialis. *Source:* Reprinted from *Procedures and Techniques in Emergency Medicine* (p 101) by RR Simon and BE Brenner with permission of the Williams & Wilkins Company, Baltimore, © 1982.

anesthetic solution. If paresthesias cannot be elicited, then instill about 5 cc of anesthetic in a fanlike fashion at the estimated location of the nerve. Take care not to injure adjacent tendons. Do not use anesthetic with epinephrine.

Ulnar Nerve Block

Anatomy

At the elbow, the ulnar nerve lies between the olecranon and the medial epicondyle, as shown in Figure 3-14.

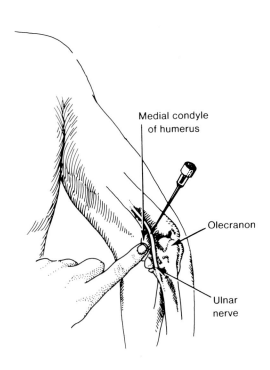

Figure 3-14 The ulnar nerve at the elbow. The posterior aspect of the elbow is pictured. Note that the nerve lies between the olecranon and the medial epicondyle. *Source:* Reprinted from *Procedures and Techniques in Emergency Medicine* (p 101) by RR Simon and BE Brenner with permission of the Williams & Wilkins Company, Baltimore, © 1982.

Five centimeters proximal to the flexor crease of the wrist the nerve divides into palmar and dorsal branches. The dorsal branch provides sensation to the dorsum of the little finger, the dorsum of the ulnar half of the ring finger, and the ulnar aspect of the dorsum of the hand. The palmar branch courses just below the flexor carpi ulnaris at the wrist, and is immediately adjacent to the ulnar artery, as shown in Figure 3-15. It provides sensation to the palmar aspects of the little finger, the palmar aspect of the ulnar half of the ring finger, and the ulnar aspect of the palm.

Blocking the ulnar nerve at the elbow provides anesthesia to the entire little finger, the ulnar half of the ring finger, and the ulnar aspects of the palm and dorsal hand. Blocking the palmar branch at the wrist anesthetizes only the palmar aspects of the little finger, the ulnar half of the ring finger, and the ulnar aspect of the palm.

Technique

To block the ulnar nerve at the elbow, first palpate the nerve between the medial epicondyle and the olecranon. Then inject about 2 cc of anesthetic on both sides of the nerve, but not into the nerve itself (Fig. 3-14).

To block the ulnar nerve (palmar branch) at the wrist, locate the flexor carpi ulnaris by having the patient ulnar deviate the wrist. Then locate the pisiform bone on the ulnar aspect of the flexor surface of the wrist. The flexor carpi ulnaris can easily be palpated at its attachment to the pisiform bone. Insert the needle perpendicular to the skin just radial to the flexor carpi ulnaris tendon at the proximal skin crease of the wrist. Attempt to induce paresthesias. Then withdraw 1 to 2 mm and inject 2 cc of anesthetic solution. If paresthesia cannot be produced, inject about 4 cc of anesthetic in a fanlike distribution at the estimated location of the nerve. Do not use anesthetic with epinephrine.

Radial Nerve Block

Anatomy

The radial nerve accompanies the radial artery in the forearm. Then about 7 cm proximal to the wrist, the nerve sends out a superficial branch which divides into several rami that provide sensation to the extensor surface of the thumb, the extensor surfaces of the proximal index and middle fingers, the extensor surface of the proximal portion of the radial half of the ring finger, as well as the radial portion of the dorsum of the hand.

Technique

Since the rami are subcutaneous at the wrist, this is the best level at which to inject. Raise a subcutaneous wheal beginning at the proximal flexor crease of the wrist ulnar to the radial artery, then spanning around the radial aspect of

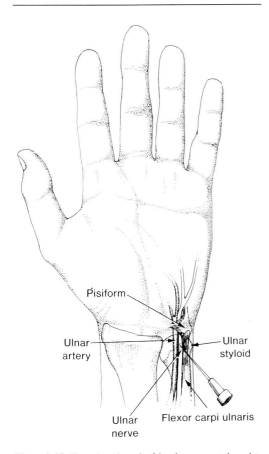

Figure 3-15 The palmar branch of the ulnar nerve at the wrist. The nerve courses next to the ulnar artery, and deep to the flexor carpi ulnaris. The nerve courses radial to the easily palpable pisiform bone. *Source:* Reprinted from *Procedures and Techniques in Emergency Medicine* (p 102) by RR Simon and BE Brenner with permission of the Williams & Wilkins Company, Baltimore, © 1982.

the wrist, and ending up about half-way across the dorsum of the wrist (Figs. 3-16 and 3-17). Do not use anesthetic with epinephrine.

Usually about 10 cc of anesthetic solution is required for a radial nerve block.

Digital Nerve Block

Anatomy

The digital nerves course along the radial and ulnar aspects of the phalanges to supply sensory innervation to the fingers, as shown in Figure 3-18.

Technique

The classic technique for the digital nerve block is to instill anesthetic on both sides of the base of the finger. Inject from the dorsal aspect, and aim toward the ventral aspect. Locate the bone with the needle, and then instill about 1 cc of anesthetic as shown in Figure 3-19.

Injecting into the finger causes local swelling, and can cause decreased local blood flow until the swelling goes down (5 to 10 minutes). The

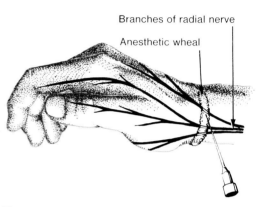

Figure 3-17 Radial nerve block. Raise a wheal around the radial aspect of the wrist, ending about halfway across the dorsum of the wrist. *Source:* Reprinted from *Procedures and Techniques in Emergency Medicine* (p 104) by RR Simon and BE Brenner with permission of the Williams & Wilkins Company, Baltimore, © 1982.

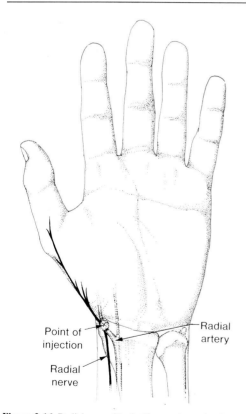

Figure 3-16 Radial nerve block. The starting point for the subcutaneous wheal is just ulnar to the radial artery pulse at the proximal crease of the wrist. *Source:* Reprinted from *Procedures and Techniques in Emergency Medicine* (p 104) by RR Simon and BE Brenner with permission of the Williams & Wilkins Company, Baltimore, © 1982.

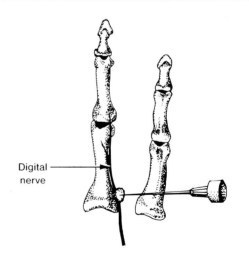

Figure 3-18 The digital nerve. The digital nerve courses immediately adjacent to the bone on both sides of the phalanges. In this illustration only one nerve is pictured. *Source:* Reprinted from *Procedures and Techniques in Emergency Medicine* (p 104) by RR Simon and BE Brenner with permission of the Williams & Wilkins Company, Baltimore, © 1982.

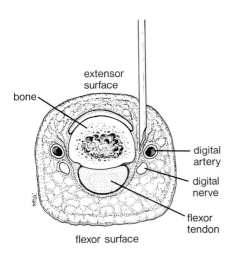

extensor
surface

bone

digital
artery

digital
nerve

flexor
tendon

flexor surface

Figure 3-19 Digital nerve block. Cross-section of the finger. Instill 1 cc of anesthetic just adjacent to, and at the ventral surface of the bone.

space technique has the advantage of not causing as much edema in the finger.

With both techniques, both sides of the finger must be injected. In some patients a wheal must also be raised over the dorsum of the finger to block the small dorsal nerves that course down the finger.

In the case of the thumb, it is necessary to raise a U-shaped wheal along the dorsum and sides of the thumb. In the case of the little finger, it is necessary to raise a wheal along the ulnar aspect of the finger.

Caution: Never use anesthetic solution mixed with epinephrine for digital nerve blocks, or local ischemia can result.

site of injection is from the dorsum of the finger, because with this approach the chances of injuring the delicate flexor tendons and tendon sheath are low.

An alternate method of blocking the digital nerve is to inject the palmar aspect of the web space with 1 to 2 cc of anesthetic on both sides of the finger, as shown in Figure 3-20. The web

SELECTED NERVE BLOCKS OF THE LOWER EXTREMITY

Posterior Tibial Nerve Block

Anatomy

The posterior tibial nerve is located between the Achilles tendon and the medial maleolus. The nerve runs alongside the posterior tibial artery (Fig. 3-21) and then branches into the

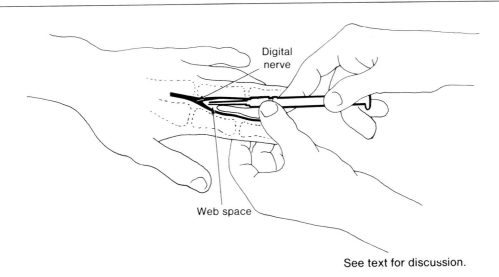

Digital
nerve

Web space

See text for discussion.

Figure 3-20 Digital nerve block, web space injection. Advance the needle 0.5 cm into the anterior aspect of the web space and instill anesthetic. The web space on both sides must be injected to obtain anesthesia for a given finger. *Source:* Reprinted from *Procedures and Techniques in Emergency Medicine* (p 105) by RR Simon and BE Brenner with permission of the Williams & Wilkins Company, Baltimore, © 1982.

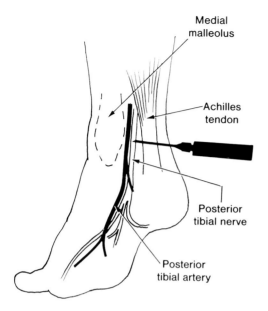

Figure 3-21 Posterior tibial nerve block. Note that the nerve runs just posterior and lateral to the posterior tibial artery, between the Achilles tendon and the medial malleolus. *Source:* Reprinted from *Procedures and Techniques in Emergency Medicine* (p 106) by RR Simon and BE Brenner with permission of the Williams & Wilkins Company, Baltimore, © 1982.

medial and lateral plantar nerves which supply sensation to the sole of the foot (Figs. 3-21 and 3-22).

Technique (Figure 3-21)

Place the patient in a prone position. Then enter the skin just lateral to the posterior tibial artery pulse, at the level of the proximal half of the medial malleolus. The needle is medial to the Achilles tendon. Advance the needle until it touches the tibia. If paresthesia occurs, pull back 1 to 2 mm and instill 5 cc of anesthetic solution. Otherwise, redirect the needle slightly medially or laterally in an attempt to produce paresthesias. If no paresthesias can be elicited, instill 10 cc of anesthesia in a fanlike distribution around the estimated location of the posterior tibial nerve. Do not use anesthetic solution with epinephrine.

Sural Nerve Block

Anatomy

The sural nerve lies between the lateral malleolus and the Achilles tendon. It supplies sensation to the heel and the lateral aspect of the foot, as shown in Figure 3-22.

Technique

Place the patient prone. Enter the skin just lateral to the Achilles tendon at the level of the

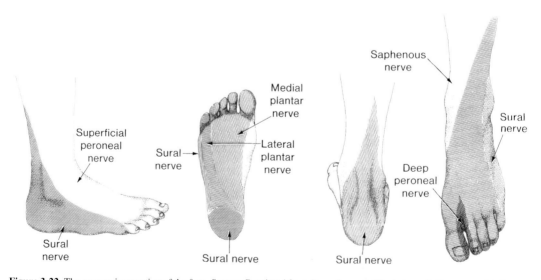

Figure 3-22 The sensory innervation of the foot. *Source:* Reprinted from *Procedures and Techniques in Emergency Medicine* (p 105) by RR Simon and BE Brenner with permission of the Williams & Wilkins Company, Baltimore, © 1982.

top of the lateral malleolus. Then instill about 5 cc of anesthetic solution in a fanlike fashion between the Achilles tendon and the lateral malleolus about ½ cm beneath the surface of the skin, as shown in Figure 3-23.

Saphenous Nerve Block

Anatomy

The saphenous nerve follows the saphenous vein across the anterior aspect of the medial malleolus. The nerve provides proximal sensation to the dorsum of the foot.

Technique

Have the patient lie supine with the foot plantar flexed. Then enter the skin just medial to the extensor hallucis longus tendon, just above the midportion of the medial malleolus. Then bur-

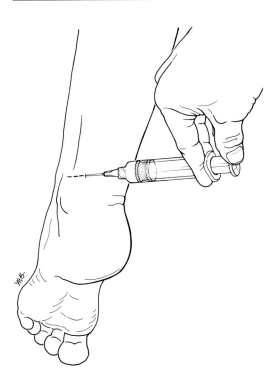

Figure 3-23 Sural nerve block. Inject 5 cc of anesthetic in the subcutaneous plane between the Achilles tendon and the lateral malleolus.

row in the subcutaneous tissue to the posterior aspect of the tibia, staying superficial to the saphenous vein. Slowly instill 3 cc of anesthetic as the needle is withdrawn (Fig. 3-24). Do not use anesthetic solution with epinephrine.

Superficial Peroneal Nerve Block

Anatomy

The superficial peroneal nerve exits the deep fascia of the lower leg just above and anterior to

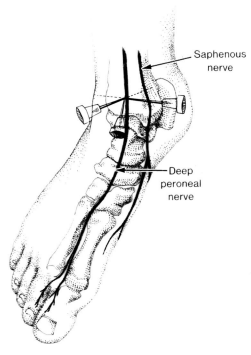

Figure 3-24 Saphenous and deep peroneal nerve block. The needle in the middle of the illustration shows the entry point through the skin. The needle in the middle can be directed posteriorly to anesthetize the deep peroneal nerve. The needle on the left-hand part of the illustration tracks medially to block the saphenous nerve. The needle on the right-hand part of the picture tracks laterally to anesthetize the cutaneous branches of the superficial peroneal nerve. The cutaneous branches themselves are not shown on this illustration. *Source:* Reprinted from *Procedures and Techniques in Emergency Medicine* (p 108) by RR Simon and BE Brenner with permission of the Williams & Wilkins Company, Baltimore, © 1982.

the lateral malleolus. The nerve then arborizes in the subcutaneous tissue to innervate the skin of the dorsum of the foot, as shown in Figure 3-22. It is the major sensory nerve to the dorsum of the foot, with the sural nerve innervating only the lateral aspect, the saphenous only the proximal aspect, and the deep peroneal only the space between the great toe and the second toe.

Technique

Enter the skin at the anterior border of the tibia at the level of the superior part of the medial malleolus. Then track laterally in the subcutaneous plane to the lateral malleolus. Slowly withdraw, instilling about 5 to 10 cc of anesthetic in the subcutaneous plane as illustrated in Figure 3-24. Note that the point of entry is the same as for the saphenous nerve block, and hence the two nerves can be blocked at the same time.

Deep Peroneal Nerve Block

Anatomy

The deep peroneal nerve passes deep to the flexor retinaculum of the ankle. It is primarily a motor nerve, but does send a small cutaneous branch to provide sensation to the region between the first and second toes, as shown in Figure 3-22.

Technique

The needle is inserted into the anterior ankle, between the medial and lateral malleoli (at the same point of entry as for the saphenous and superficial peroneal nerve blocks). The needle is inserted directly posteriorly until it hits the tibia. Then 3 to 4 cc of anesthetic solution is instilled, as shown in Figure 3-24. Do not use anesthetic solution with epinephrine. This block is frequently unsuccessful, however, anesthesia is easily obtained with local infiltration between the first and second toes.

Digital Nerve Blocks in the Foot

Anatomy

The digital nerves run along the medial and lateral phalanges of the toes, and provide sensation to the toes.

The great toe, in addition, receives sensation from small, superficial cutaneous nerves.

Technique

For toes other than the great toe, the skin can be entered at a single point over the dorsum of the base of the toe in the midline, as shown in Figure 3-25. The needle is then directed first

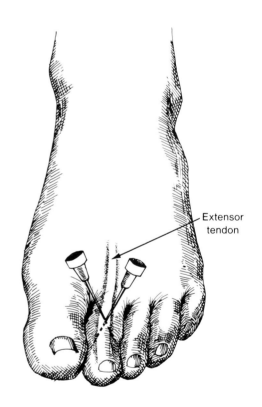

Extensor tendon

Figure 3-25 Digital nerve block of toes 2 to 5. The needle enters the skin in the midline, and then is directed first to one side and then the other side of the toe. *Source:* Reprinted from *Procedures and Techniques in Emergency Medicine* (p 109) by RR Simon and BE Brenner with permission of the Williams & Wilkins Company, Baltimore, © 1982.

along one side of the bone to the plantar aspect of that bone, and then 1 cc of anesthetic is instilled. The same process is then performed on the other side.

For the great toe a subcutaneous circle of anesthesia around the base of the toe is required in addition to the digital nerve block. Begin by entering the extensor surface of the lateral aspect of the base of the toe (point A in Fig. 3-26).

First, pass the needle directly down alongside the bone, and instill 2 cc of anesthetic at the plantar aspect of the bone, to block the digital nerve. Then redirect the needle over the dorsum of the toe, and instill 2 cc of anesthetic into the subcutaneous plane to block the small cutaneous nerves. Next enter at point B in Figure 3-26, and instill 2 cc of anesthetic at the plantar aspect of the bone on the medial side, as well as 1 cc into the subcutaneous tissue of the medial aspect of the toe. Finally, inject 1 to 2 cc into the sub-cutaneous tissue at the plantar aspect of the toe. Allow approximately 10 minutes for the anes-thetic to diffuse before suturing or debriding.

Do not use anesthetic with epinephrine for digital blocks of the foot; ischemic necrosis can result.

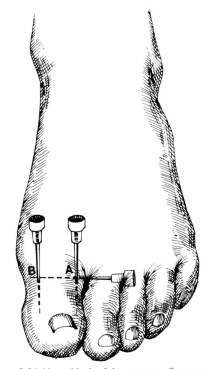

Figure 3-26 Nerve block of the great toe. See text, Deep Peroneal Nerve Block, for discussion. *Source:* Reprinted from *Procedures and Techniques in Emergency Medicine* (p 108) by RR Simon and BE Brenner with permission of the Williams & Wilkins Company, Baltimore, © 1982.

.

Chapter 4

Precare: Patient Evaluation, Hemostasis Techniques, and Wound Cleansing and Antisepsis

The precare of the patient with a wound begins with a general evaluation of the patient, including history of how the wound occurred, of medications and associated illnesses, and of tetanus immunization status. Hemostasis must be gained if there is active hemorrhaging.

Proper wound cleansing and preparation significantly decrease the incidence of infection in lacerations. High-pressure irrigation removes bacteria and foreign material from wounds significantly better than low-pressure irrigation. Topical povidone-iodine solution decreases the wound infection rate without causing tissue necrosis. Detergent agents, however, raise the rate of wound sepsis and cause focal tissue necrosis.

PATIENT EVALUATION

General Evaluation
(see also Chapter 8)

The care of the patient as a whole takes precedence over treatment of the local wounds. The physician must be sure that the airway is secure and that there are no cervical spine injuries. Next ventilation should be assessed and the patient checked for adequacy of circulation. Any bleeding from wounds should be immediately con-

trolled with local pressure (see Hemostasis, below).

The patient should be questioned about a past history of illnesses, present medications, and allergies (particularly in regard to local anesthetics and antibiotics). The physician should investigate whether a serious medical or psychological disorder may have led to the wound. For example, did the scalp laceration result from a fall during a Stokes-Adams attack? Was the laceration self-induced? Also, the physician should determine whether conditions exist that will impair healing, such as diabetes, peripheral vascular disease, or chronic use of corticosteroids.

Tetanus Prophylaxis

Determine if the patient is up to date on tetanus immunizations. Remember that a patient who has not received an adequate primary immunization series must be treated with both tetanus toxoid and tetanus immune globulin (Table 4-1).

HEMOSTASIS

The basic maneuver to stop bleeding is to apply pressure over the wound for 10 to 20 min-

Table 4-1 Guidelines for Tetanus Prophylaxis

Tetanus Toxoid Immunizations	Wound Type[a]	Tetanus Toxoid	Tetanus Immune Globulin
Three or more, last within 5 yr	Clean, minor	No	No
Three or more, last within 5 yr	Significant	No	No
Three or more, last within 10 yr	Clean, minor	No	No
Three or more, last within 10 yr	Significant	Yes	No
Three or more, last > 10 yr	Clean, minor	Yes	No
Three or more, last > 10 yr	Significant	Yes	No
Unknown or < three	Clean, minor	Yes	No
Unknown or < three	Significant	Yes	Yes

[a]Clean, minor = clean, superficial wounds. Significant = contaminated wounds, punctures, burns, frostbite, crush injuries, suturable lacerations. (Based on recommendations in MMWR Vol. 34, p. 422, July 12, 1985. Check current MMWR for possible updates in recommendations for tetanus prophylaxis.)

utes. Direct pressure is superior to the use of tourniquets, because the blood flow to noninjured tissue is not cut off, as occurs with tourniquets. Before applying local pressure, all clots should be irrigated from the wound.

Axiom: Direct pressure is the method of choice for controlling wound hemorrhage.

In the majority of patients, local pressure and elevation are all that is needed to control hemorrhage.

In problem wounds, where hemorrhaging persists despite local pressure, several maneuvers are available to stop bleeding. The first is a trial of topical epinephrine. Dilute 1 cc of epinephrine 1:1,000 (= 1 mg), in 4 to 5 cc of sterile saline. Soak a 4 inch × 4 inch piece of gauze in this solution, and then hold the gauze over the bleeding region for 5 minutes. This procedure will adequately control most small, dermal bleeding. Because the vasoconstriction is temporary, larger vessels will need to be ligated at the time of definitive repair. Epinephrine is contraindicated in regions such as the fingers and toes, the tip of the nose, and the penis, where ischemic necrosis can occur secondary to constric-

tion of essential arteries. Epinephrine must be used with caution in patients with a history of coronary artery disease or cardiac dysrhythmias. When epinephrine is contraindicated, packing the wound with Gelfoam and then applying constant pressure will often control bleeding.

In highly vascular regions such as the face and scalp, which continue to ooze blood, perhaps the easiest and most effective way to control bleeding is to suture the wound closed. The intrinsic pressure inside the suture loop is enough to tamponade small bleeders.

Persistently bleeding small vessels can be clamped and then ligated. However, never clamp and ligate bleeding arteries in the wrist and hand, or any major arteries anywhere in the body. Maintain hemostasis with local pressure and then check with a consultant concerning possible microsurgical reanastomosis.

HAIR REMOVAL

In one study, shaving the skin prior to elective surgery led to a 5.6 percent infection rate, compared to 0.6 percent when the skin was prepared with a depilatory.[163] This potentiation of infection is most marked when shaving is performed 24 hours prior to a planned surgery. However, shaving has not been shown to increase the infection rate in wounds sutured in the emergency department.

Eyebrows should never be shaved or clipped. Eyebrows are slow to grow back once removed. In addition, eyebrows serve as valuable landmarks for wound repair.

Axiom: Never shave the eyebrows.

IRRIGATION

Irrigation is the time-honored method for removing bacteria and dirt from wounds.

Because it does not irritate body tissues, normal saline is the irrigation fluid of choice. Various other solutions cause varying degrees of tissue damage (see Topical Antiseptics and Surface Active Agents, below). Specifically, detergents or alcohols should *never* be used in or near an open wound.

The efficacy of an irrigation system in removing foreign material from a wound is directly related to the force of the irrigant stream and the surface area (size) of the particles being removed. Hence, larger particles are more easily removed from a wound than smaller particles, and high-pressure irrigation is more efficient than low-pressure irrigation.

Axiom: Large particles are more easily removed from a wound than small particles. High-pressure irrigation is more effective than low-pressure irrigation.

Hence vigorous irrigation is necessary to remove very small particles, such as bacteria.

Irrigation using a bulb or asepto syringe generates relatively low pressures, on the order of only 0.05 psi. Irrigation using a 35-cc syringe and a 19-gauge needle generates intermediate pressures, on the order of 8 psi.[188] Irrigation using a mechanical jet device generates high pressures, on the order of 80 psi. In laboratory animals with contaminated lacerations, intermediate and high-pressure irrigation are superior to low-pressure irrigation in decreasing the wound infection rate.[19,85,90,152,173] Inter-

estingly, however, the 80-psi jet is probably not superior to the 8-psi 35-cc syringe technique.[188]

Although high-pressure irrigation decreases wound bacterial contamination, the technique has its side effects. In one study, with the high-pressure jet (70 psi), irrigation solution dissected laterally 14 mm from the wound edge, and deeply, 3 mm below the base of the wound.[188] With the 35-cc syringe and 19-gauge needle (8 psi), the irrigation solution spread laterally only 3 mm, and there was no appreciable deep spread.[188] However, neither technique caused the deep or lateral spread of bacteria that had been swabbed on top of the wounds.[188] Because of the potential for lateral spread and subsequent systemic absorption, only normal saline or Ringer's lactate should be used for high-pressure irrigation.

Uncontaminated wounds irrigated with either the high-pressure jet or syringe technique, and then subsequently contaminated with *Staphylococcus aureus* develop significantly more wound infections than control wounds that are not irrigated under pressure.[188]

Note: Use only normal saline or Ringer's lactate for high-pressure irrigation.

To summarize the experimental data, high-pressure irrigation is more effective than low-pressure irrigation in removing bacteria and foreign material from contaminated wounds. However, in uncontaminated wounds, tissue damage caused by high-pressure irrigation may actually increase the risk of infection.

Therefore, for clean, uncontaminated wounds (such as a shear laceration caused by a clean knife blade) the authors recommend the use of low-pressure irrigation, using either a bulb syringe or a standard 35-cc syringe fitted with an 18-gauge needle, but depressing gently on the plunger. For contaminated wounds we recommend using a 35-cc syringe fitted with either an 18-gauge angiocath or a 19-gauge needle, and depressing the plunger with full force. Contaminated wounds cannot be adequately cleansed by attaching intravenous tubing to a bag of normal saline, and irrigating under the force of gravity.

When performing the high-pressure syringe irrigation, keep the tip of the catheter 3–4 mm above the wound surface to avoid ballooning up the deep tissue planes with saline.

The volume of fluid needed for irrigation will vary according to the size of the wound and the degree of contamination. A 2- to 4-cm wound can be adequately cleansed with 250 cc. Larger volumes are required for larger wounds.

TOPICAL ANTISEPTICS AND SURFACE ACTIVE AGENTS

Wound preparation does not end with irrigation. Proper antiseptics can aid in wound healing. A topical agent should promote wound antisepsis without damaging tissue. Much controversy exists as to which, if any, of these agents should be employed.

Tissue Damage of Topical Agents

Table 4-2 lists various topical agents, along with their relative toxicities when applied to open wounds.

Isopropyl alcohol is the most damaging agent. In one histologic study, alcohol essentially fixed the tissues, causing necrosis of all elements.[16]

Following isopropyl alcohol, detergents are the next most toxic substance to the subcutaneous tissues. Detergents are designed for cleaning intact skin prior to elective surgery, or for cleaning the surgeon's hands; their use in open lacerations can have disastrous effects. For example, in one study, hexachlorophene and

---

Table 4-2 Toxicity of Topical Agents.*

Saline = 0
Pluronic F-68 = 0
Betadine prep solution
  (povidone-iodine solution) = 1+
Hexachlorophene solution = 2+
Quaternary ammonia solution = 3+
Hydrogen pyroxide = 6+
Betadine surgical scrub
  (povidone-iodine and detergent) = 8+
Phisohex
  (Hexachlorophene and detergent) = 8+
Isopropyl alcohol = 10+

*Saline (0) is the standard. The higher the number, the more caustic the agent.[1–4]

---

povidone-iodine *aqueous solutions* caused little or no damage to cartilage and soft tissue when injected directly into the knee joints of laboratory animals.[62] However, these same agents in a *detergent base* (Phisohex and Betadine surgical scrub) caused widespread tissue necrosis, as well as ankylosis of the joints.

In another study, povidone-iodine solution (Betadine Prep) led to a significant decrease in the infection rate when applied to open wounds, while povidone-iodine in a detergent base (Betadine Scrub) applied to the same wounds actually led to an increase in the rate of infection compared to control animals.[38] Therefore, no topical agent containing a detergent base should be used in or even near an open wound.

Axiom: No topical agent containing a detergent should ever be used on an open wound.

Aqueous hydrogen pyroxide, although commonly used to clean open wounds, can have damaging effects. In one study of wound histology following the application of various agents, pyroxide was found to cause almost complete blockage of the microvasculature.[16] Furthermore, peroxide is a relatively poor antibacterial agent.[145] Although peroxide is useful for cleaning off blood from intact skin and laboratory coats, it should not be applied to open wounds.

Pluronic F-68, a relatively new surface active agent, is remarkably nontoxic.[151] However, this agent does not kill bacteria.

Povidone-iodine solution is a superb antiseptic, with relatively few toxic effects. We feel that povidone-iodine is the antiseptic solution of choice for use in the emergency department.

Axiom: Povidone-iodine prep solution is the antiseptic of choice for use in the emergency department.

Povidone-Iodine Solution

Elemental iodine in solution is unstable, and has only a short-lived antimicrobial effect when applied to tissues. Iodine bound to the povidone carrier is far more stable, and has a much more sustained antibacterial effect when applied to the tissues. In a 10 percent povidone-iodine solution, approximately 90 percent of the iodine is bound to povidone, and the remaining 10 percent is free (active) iodine. There is some evidence that because of peculiarities in the dissociation kinetics of povidone-iodine, a 1 percent povidone-iodine solution may contain as much free iodine as a 10 percent solution.[9]

The antibacterial range of povidone iodine includes *Staphylococcus aureus, Streptococcus pyogenes, Streptococcus viridans, Klebsiella, Pseudomonas, Proteus,* and *Escherichia coli.*[102,159] Interestingly, a 1 percent povidone-iodine solution appears to be as effective as the stock 10 percent solution in killing bacteria, possibly due to the relatively high amount of free iodine present in the 1 percent solution.[9] Emergence of bacterial strains resistant to povidone-iodine has not been shown to occur in laboratory studies.[102]

Several human studies demonstrate the efficacy of povidone-iodine (applied directly to the open wound just prior to closure) in decreasing the incidence of surgical wound infections. In one of the initial studies, in which wounds were treated with either aerosolized 5 percent povidone-iodine or an inert powder, Gilmore and associates demonstrated an infection rate of 9 percent in the control group, versus 0 percent in the povidone group.[76] In a study of abdominal surgical wounds, many of which were grossly contaminated, Gilmore and Sanderson documented an infection rate of 24 percent in the control group, compared to 8.6 percent in those treated with povidone-iodine.[75] In both these studies the povidone-iodine was applied only after the deep tissues (including the peritoneum) had been closed. In a prospective, randomly assigned trial, Sindelar and Mason demonstrated that a 60-second irrigation with a 10 percent povidone-iodine solution decreased the postoperative infection rate from 15.1 to 2.9 percent.[169]

Not all studies show a benefit from povidone-iodine, however. Viljanto, in a study of children undergoing appendectomy, found a significant decrease in the infection rate in those treated with a 1 percent povidone-iodine solution versus control subjects, but an increased infection rate in those treated with a 5 percent aerosolized spray.[185]

Of interest to the emergency specialist, there are initial reports that treating emergency department wounds with povidone-iodine significantly decreases the rate of wound infection.[137,196]

Local reactions to povidone are rare. In one study of 500 patients who had povidone-iodine applied to open surgical wounds, there were no allergic or other local reactions, and no systemic effects on serum iodine or thyroxine levels.[169] Povidone-iodine does appear to affect in vitro granulocyte migration.[185]

Some authors have brought up the theoretical possibility of povidone-iodine disrupting the healing process.[52,145] However, in animal studies there has been no difference in wound histology or tensile strength between the povidone-iodine treated group and the control group.[76,151]

Apart from allergic reactions and theoretical alterations of white cell function, the main side effects appear to be in terms of thyroid function tests. Investigators have demonstrated a rise in thyroid-stimulating hormone (TSH), but with preservation of total T4 in women using povidone-iodine as a daily douche.[116,156] Infants born to mothers using the daily douches have had transient depressions of the serum thyroxine.[116]

In summary, topical povidone-iodine appears to be an effective, and relatively nontoxic topical antiseptic solution. The authors recommend diluting the stock 10 percent solution 1:10 with saline to yield a 1 percent solution. The fascia should first be closed, and then the dilute solution applied with a 4 inch × 4 inch gauze pad directly to the wound itself for approximately 1 minute. The solution should not be irrigated off prior to final wound closure.

TOPICAL ANTIBIOTICS

Topical antibiotics, especially ampicillin and kanamycin, have been shown to be effective in decreasing infection rates in operative wounds.[77] There has not been an extensive experience in the use of topical antibiotics for traumatic lacerations. We do not recommend topical antibiotics for general use in the emergency department because of the possibility of skin sensitization, and of selecting resistant strains of bacteria. However, topical antibiotics may be useful for contaminated wounds when povidone-iodine is contraindicated.

Chapter 5

Basic Laceration Repair

This chapter outlines first the basic principles, and then the techniques of basic laceration repair. The first part of the chapter starts with a discussion of closure by primary, secondary, and tertiary intent. Next, the concepts of wound tension and wound edge eversion are presented. The second part of the chapter deals with the basic techniques of wound closure, beginning with débridement and undermining, and ending with basic suturing techniques and the use of nonsuture adjuncts to skin closure.

BASIC PRINCIPLES OF LACERATION REPAIR

Categories of Wound Closure

Closure by Primary Intent

Closure by primary intent occurs when the wound is repaired without delay following the injury, prior to the formation of granulation tissue. Closure may be with sutures, skin tapes, staples, or tissue adhesives. Primary closure yields the fastest healing and generally speaking the best cosmetic result.

Primary closure is the treatment of choice for repairing any wound that is not infected or grossly contaminated. Time is an important factor in wounds that are closed by primary intent. As one might expect, the potential for infection

increases as the period of time from injury to repair lengthens. Time allows bacteria to multiply, and the wound infection rate is directly proportional to the number of bacteria present.

Most lacerations can be closed within 8 hours from the time of injury. Every injury must be treated on an individual basis, however. For example, clean shear facial lacerations can be closed safely within 24 hours of the injury because of the excellent vasculature existing in this region. Similarly, uncontaminated, shear lacerations of the extremities can often be closed within 12 hours. However, the maximum time to primary repair should be reduced by as much as half where there is, for example, a debilitated host, poor regional perfusion (such as with peripheral vascular disease or a flap laceration), lacerations due to crushing injuries, or grossly contaminated wounds. Patients should be warned of the increased infection potential caused by the delay in repair.

In busy emergency departments there is frequently a delay before a patient with a laceration can be evaluated by the physician. In such instances a nurse or technician should irrigate the laceration with saline, apply a 1 percent solution of povidone-iodine, and cover the region with a sterile dressing.

Closure by Secondary Intent

Healing by secondary intent occurs when the wound is allowed to granulate on its own, without surgical closure. The tissue is cleaned and prepped in the usual manner and the wound is covered with a sterile dressing. Secondary intent is the procedure of choice for closing certain defects. For example, fingertip amputations allowed to heal by secondary intent generally speaking yield better cosmetic and functional results than those closed by primary intent (see Chapter 8). In addition, partial-thickness tissue losses are best left to heal on their own without grafting or other specific intervention.

Closure by Tertiary Intent (Delayed Primary Closure)

Healing by tertiary intent means that the wound is initially cleaned and dressed, as with secondary intent, but then the patient returns in 3 to 4 days for definitive closure. Another name for this technique is *delayed primary closure* (see Chapter 7). This is the method of choice for repairing contaminated lacerations that would leave unacceptable scars if not closed. Examples include most mammalian bites to the hand, contaminated crush-lacerations, and cases in which the patient has delayed too long for the wound to be closed by primary intent. For example, an alcoholic who falls and lacerates his arm but delays 24 hours before seeking help can still have the wound repaired by delayed primary closure. Often the final cosmetic result with closure by tertiary intent is identical to the result that would have been obtained with closure by primary intent.

In summary, to quote Dr. Peter Rosen: "If a wound is dirty, it shouldn't be closed; and if it's clean, it cannot be left open."[195]

Skin Tension Lines

A knowledge of the body's normal skin tension lines is important in the management of lacerations. The skin tension lines are the creases that naturally appear when the skin is gathered together between two fingers, as illustrated in Figure 5-1. The usual pattern of the body's skin tension lines is pictured in Figure 5-2.

Lacerations that run parallel to the skin tension lines leave less noticeable scars than those that run perpendicular. Thus a forehead laceration that runs up and down, from brow to scalp line, will heal with more scarring than one that runs parallel to the furrow line, as shown in Figure 5-3.

In addition, lacerations that run parallel to the flexor creases of joints are much less prone to lead to skin contractures than those that run perpendicular. Thus a flexion contracture is much more likely to occur with a finger laceration that runs perpendicular to an interphalangeal flexion crease than with one that runs parallel to the crease.

Skin tension lines become important during débridement, because tissue should be excised in such a manner as to make the final scar line up with the natural skin creases. Plastic surgeons utilize the concept of skin tension lines during scar revisions, realigning scars to run parallel to the normal tension lines.

Wound Edge Eversion and Inversion

Another important concept in wound repair is *wound edge eversion*. In a properly sutured

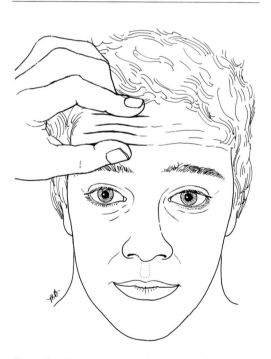

Figure 5-1 Gathering the skin between two fingers brings out the normal skin tension lines for an area.

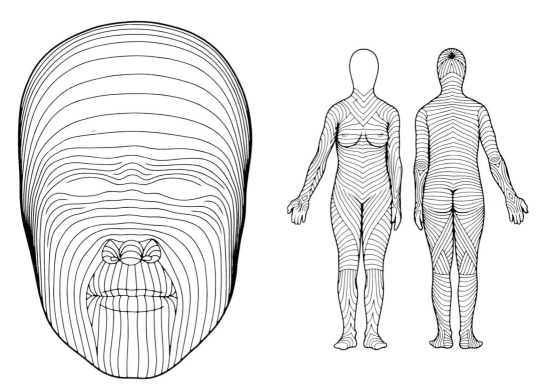

Figure 5-2 These figures illustrate the basic pattern of the body's skin tension lines. There is, of course, a fair amount of variation from person to person. *Source:* Reprinted from *Procedures and Techniques in Emergency Medicine* (p 280) by RR Simon and BE Brenner with permission of the Williams & Wilkins Company, Baltimore, © 1982.

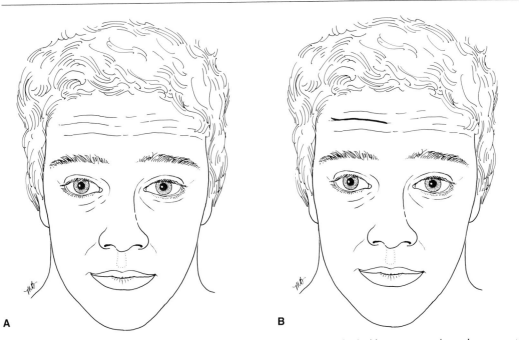

A   B

Figure 5-3 The scar that runs perpendicular to the skin tension lines (**A**) tends to heal with more contraction and consequent distortion of the facial features than the scar that runs parallel to the natural tension lines (**B**).

laceration, the wound edges should be slightly everted, or at the least made level with the plane of the tissue. The edges should not be allowed to invert. (Fig. 5-4.)

The advantages of everted edges are many. First, epithelialization occurs twice as rapidly than as with inverted edges. As illustrated in Figure 5-4, the epidermoid cells directly abut when the wound edges are everted; but do not come into contact when the wound edges are inverted. Second, because of the rapid formation of an epithelial barrier, the rate of wound infection is decreased. Last and probably most important, wounds with everted edges heal in such a way that the final scar is flat, and less noticeable than the deeply ridged scars that occur as the result of wound edge inversion.

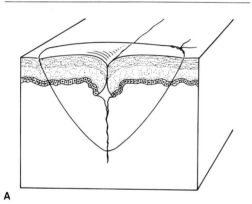

A

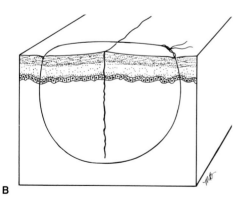

B

Figure 5-4 A. The base of the loop is not broad enough, and consequently there is inversion of the wound edges. Notice how basal, regenerative epidermal cells on either side of the wound do not come into contact, thus delaying the healing. **B.** There is a broad base to the suture loop, and consequently the edges evert. Notice that in this instance the basal epidermal cells do come into contact, thus facilitating healing.

Wound Tension

Extrinsic Tension

The *extrinsic tension* equals the force with which the wound edges tend to pull apart (Fig. 5-5). In cases where the wound edges tend to come together even before the placement of sutures, such as the web spaces of the fingers, the extrinsic tension is negligible. Conversely, in instances where the wound edges gape far apart, such as lacerations on the lower leg and lacerations involving the actual avulsion of tissue, the extrinsic tension pulling against the sutures is great. The extrinsic tension pulling at any given suture varies inversely with the total number of sutures used per centimeter. Just as there is half as much tension per rope if ten as opposed to five ropes are used to suspend a weight, in like manner there is less extrinsic tension per suture if ten as opposed to five suture loops are used to close a given laceration. The greater the extrinsic tension at any given suture, the greater the tendency for the suture to rip the tissue, and thus the greater the tendency for unsightly suture marks once the wound has healed (see Suture Marks, below).

In gaping lacerations, the physician should attempt to decrease the tension with which the skin edges pull away from one another. The two

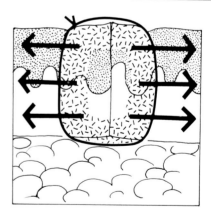

Figure 5-5 The external tension equals the force that pulls the wound edges apart. Generally speaking, the greater the initial gape of the wound, the greater the extrinsic tension when the wound is repaired. *Source:* Reprinted from *Procedures and Techniques in Emergency Medicine* (p 284) by RR Simon and BE Brenner with permission of the Williams & Wilkins Company, Baltimore, © 1982.

simplest means of achieving this decreased tension are to adequately undermine the wound, and to close the deep tissues prior to closing the skin (see Undermining, below). If these two methods fail, more complicated techniques such as advancement flaps or skin grafts are required (see Chapter 7).

Intrinsic Wound Tension

The intrinsic tension equals the pressure with which the tissues within the suture loop are squeezed together (Fig. 5-6). In wounds sutured tightly, the intrinsic tension within the suture loop is great. Conversely, when the sutures are secured with minimal force, the intrinsic tension is also minimal. During the first 48 hours of healing the intrinsic pressure within a suture loop tends to increase as the result of edema.

One of the major tenets of proper suturing technique is to cinch down on the sutures just enough to bring the skin edges into apposition, but no more. To quote a popular adage: "The wound edges should be *approximated*, and not *strangulated*." If a wound is sutured closed too tightly, perfusion to the tissue within the loop will be comprised. If this vascular compromise is enough, the tissue will actually necrose, markedly delaying healing, increasing the wound infection rate, and resulting in a much thicker scar.

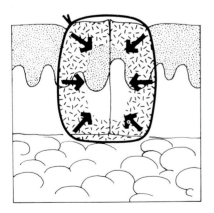

Figure 5-6 Intrinsic tension. The intrinsic tension equals the force with which the tissues within the suture loop are squeezed together. The more tightly the sutures are cinched, the greater the intrinsic tension. *Source:* Reprinted from *Procedures and Techniques in Emergency Medicine* (p 282) by RR Simon and BE Brenner with permission of the Williams & Wilkins Company, Baltimore, © 1982.

In such instances, the wound would have probably healed better if no suturing had been done.

Axiom: *It is better not to suture closed a wound at all than to suture it closed with too much tension.*

Suture Marks

Suture marks are the unsightly remnants of epithelialization down the subcutaneous tracks of skin sutures. If sutures are left in the skin for too long a period, these suture marks will become permanent. Permanent tracks can form on the face in as little as 5 days, particularly in children. In slower-healing regions of the body, such as the distal extremities, permanent marks take a minimum of one week to form.

Suture marks become more prominent with increasing extrinsic tension per suture. Thus, careful undermining helps to decrease marking. In addition, the greater the number of sutures used to close a given wound, the less the tension on each stitch, and hence the less the tendency for suture marks.

In summary, to avoid suture marks, close wounds under as little tension as possible; use an adequate number of sutures per centimeter, and insure that the patient returns for suture removal at the recommended time.

Buried Sutures

General

Closure of the deep tissue prior to closure of the skin improves the final appearance of the wound. Failure to close the deep tissues can cause unsightly shallow depressions to form as the wound heals (Fig. 5-7).

Deep sutures retard the tendency for scars to widen following the removal of the skin sutures. Further, with some facial lacerations, there is distortion in the lines of facial expression if the deep layer containing the muscles of facial expression is not repaired. Deep sutures also improve the final appearance of the wound by decreasing the tension on the skin ties, thus decreasing the suture marks.

The frequently held notion that deep sutures help reduce the incidence of wound infection by

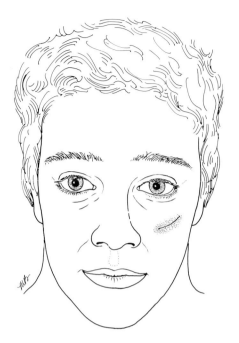

Figure 5-7 Notice the shallow depression in the region of the healed scar, caused because the deep tissues were not brought together with buried sutures during the initial repair. Although the scar itself is faint, the depression causes a final result that is noncosmetic.

eliminating the dead space, is not true. In fact, exactly the opposite appears to be the case. In experimental models the use of deep sutures actually increases the risk of infection.[52] This potentiation of wound infection is most likely the result of the foreign material serving as a nidus for infection. If one wishes to suppress the accumulation of fluid in a potentially contaminated wound, probably the best method is with the application of a pressure dressing.

Surgical Drains

Surgical drains are also often purported to decrease the rate of infection in deep lacerations. However, in controlled studies drains actually increase the rate of wound infection.[52] Therefore, drains are not advisable in the care of most lacerations sutured in the emergency department. Drains do have a role in the care of operative wounds, which is to alert the surgeon to the development of hemorrhage or abscess in deep cavities.

BASIC TECHNIQUES IN WOUND CLOSURE

Wound Débridement and Excision

There are four major indications for the excision of tissue from a wound: the removal of adherent foreign material, the trimming of irregular wound edges, the improvement of the final configuration of the wound, and the débridement of dead tissue.

Débridement of Adherent Material

Indications. Following irrigation (see Chapter 4), wounds should be carefully explored for any adherent or retained foreign material. In lacerations following falls from bicycles or motorcycles, for example, particles of dirt, gravel, and grease often become imbedded in the tissue. Such material both serves as a nidus for infection and, if close to the surface, leads to tattooing of the skin. Therefore foreign material must be eliminated.

Note: *Retained foreign material can lead to tattooing of the skin.*

Technique. The simplest means of removing adherent dirt and grease is to repeatedly abrade the soiled region with a 4 inch × 4 inch piece of gauze moistened in saline. If this fails, then one must actually excise the soiled tissue using a forceps and an iris scissors or scalpel, as shown in Figure 5-8.

Trimming the Wound Edge

Even in linear lacerations, minute irregularities are often present along the skin edge. Trimming a small amount of tissue from the wound edge takes little time and often greatly improves the final appearance after healing. Frequently only 1 mm of tissue needs to be trimmed off. The authors recommend using a sharp iris scissors, either curved or straight, depending on the wound configuration, to carefully trim off minor irregularities from the edges, as shown in Figure 5-9. A scalpel can also be used.

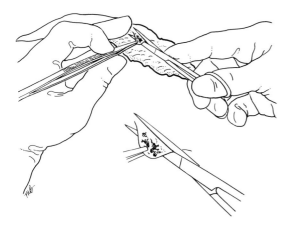

Figure 5-8 A forceps and iris scissors are employed to remove small bits of dirt that were not removed with saline irrigation or by abrading the area with moistened gauze. As little tissue as possible is excised along with the particles of dirt.

Excisions to Improve the Wound Configuration

Indications. There are several instances in which the configuration of a laceration should be altered by the physician prior to closing the wound. For example, small circular defects heal best if first converted to an ellipse by excising adjacent tissue, as will be discussed in Chapter 7.

Most wounds with multiple small irregularities can be converted into a simple ellipse prior to closure, as shown in Figure 5-10. Since irregular wounds are most commonly due to compression insults, the tissue that is excised is often crushed or devitalized. Hence the excision will not only improve the final cosmetic appearance, but also may decrease the risk of infection.

Technique. Whenever possible, plan the excision in such a way as to make the final scar conform to the skin tension lines. It is often useful to mark the pattern to be excised with a sterile skin pencil.

Excise so the final wound edge is beveled at approximately 90 degrees to the plane of the skin (Fig. 5-11A). Although some authors have recommended beveling the edge so that the tissue at the top of the wound overhangs the

tissue at the bottom (Figure 5-11B), we have not found this necessary.

When excising wound edges in regions with hair, match the angle of excision with the angle at which the hairs grow, as shown in Figure 8-6.

There are three basic means of excising the skin: using a no. 15 scalpel, using a no. 11 scalpel, and using an iris scissors.

The No. 15 Blade Technique. Grasp the skin edge with an adson forceps or skin hook and then, holding the no. 15 blade like a pencil, excise the pattern. The sharpest cutting edge of the blade is on the distal third. Use forceps only to hold the skin in place. Pulling too hard on the forceps during débridement distorts the tissue. The no. 15 blade is especially useful in creating ellipses and curves, as shown in Figure 5-12. We feel that it is the method of choice for most excisions performed in the emergency department.

The No. 11 Blade Technique. The no. 11 blade can be used to make multiple punctures along the pattern to be excised. The excision is then completed using either an iris scissors or a no. 15 scapel blade, taking care to avoid causing irregularities along the edge during excision. This technique is useful for complex lacerations (Fig. 5-13).

The Iris Scissors Technique. The wound edge is grasped with the adson forceps, as with

---

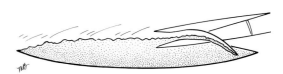

Figure 5-9 The iris scissors is used to trim away small irregularities in the edges. The bottom edge has already been trimmed in this illustration. The amount of tissue being excised is slightly exaggerated for illustrative purposes.

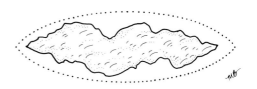

Figure 5-10 The dotted lines indicate the pattern of excision that must be followed to convert this irregular contour into a simple ellipse.

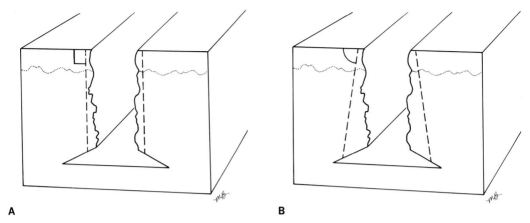

A   **B**

Figure 5-11 Wound edge excision. **A** demonstrates excision (dotted line) at 90° to the surface. **B** demonstrates excision such that the superficial portion of the wound edge overhangs the deeper portion. See text for details.

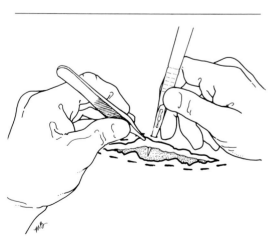

Figure 5-12 Wound edge excision using a no. 15 scalpel blade. Note that the scalpel is held like a pen.

the other two techniques, and the pattern is cut out, as shown in Figure 5-14.

Some authorities feel that a scapel is superior to scissors for trimming wound edges, because it offers less potential for crushing the tissues. However, we have generally found the final results to be indistinguishable.

Débridement of Necrotic Tissue

Indications. Tissue that is obviously necrotic should be excised prior to closure. Necrotic tissue increases the rate of wound infection and abscess formation. One must use caution, however. Tissue that has borderline viability should be left intact in areas such as the nose and the ear,

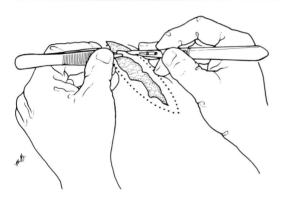

Figure 5-13 Wound edge excision using a no. 11 scalpel blade. Note that the scalpel is used to make numerous stabs (dashed lines) to mark the desired pattern. See text for details.

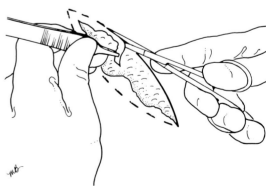

Figure 5-14 Wound edge excision using an iris scissors. In this illustration the iris scissors are cutting out a pattern already marked out by the no. 11 scalpel blade, as described in Figure 5-13.

where there is excellent vascularity, and where loss of even small amounts of tissue is often noticeable.

Technique. The technique for debriding necrotic tissue is identical with the method described above for excising tissue to improve the wound configuration.

Undermining

General Principles

As mentioned above, the principal means of decreasing extrinsic tension on a gaping wound is to undermine the tissue prior to closure. In so doing, the physician takes advantage of the skin's natural elasticity. Undermining relaxes the bonds between the subcutaneous tissue and the dermis, permitting the skin to stretch. Thus the wound edges pull together under less tension. Undermining does cause trauma to the tissues being repaired. However, the benefit of being able to approximate the tissues without undue force outweighs the ill effects of the trauma caused by the undermining itself.

Technique

In most wounds, undermining should be undertaken in the plane of the subcutaneous fat or fascia. Because the natural planes vary in different parts of the body, the exact planes will vary from region to region. For example, in the forearm the dermis is naturally separated from the underlying muscle sheaths, and therefore the subdermal fascia is the best plane in which to undermine. On the trunk, the subcutaneous fat is the best plane for undermining. In some areas undermining is difficult, such as the sole of the foot.

The extent to which the tissue is undermined depends on the extent to which the wound gapes. As a general rule, undermine to a width equal to the gape of the wound (Figure 5-15).

The easiest method of undermining is to bluntly dissect the tissues using a straight mosquito clamp with the blades initially closed. Alternatively, an iris scissors can be used. Once the tissue plane has been entered to the desired extent, spread open the blades of the scissors

(see Fig. 5-15). This process is then repeated until the entire wound has been undermined, taking care to keep undermining superficial to any important nerves, arteries, and tendons.

Some authors recommend sharp dissection with a no. 15 scalpel blade. We prefer blunt dissection in most cases, because the risk of severing vital structures is far less. One exception to this rule is shallow undermining in the dermis itself. The scalpel is then used to undermine to a depth of about 5 mm. Evert the edges so that the base of the region being cut is always in full view. Keeping the base in view decreases the chances of inadvertently severing any nerves, arteries, or tendons. However, if the tissues can be sutured easily without dermal undermining, this should be done.

The Simple Skin Suture

Choice of Materials (See Chapter 2)

Suture Material. (See Table 8-1, Chapter 8.) Choose the thinnest possible suture that will do the job. In the emergency department setting, choose either nylon or prolene for skin sutures. These materials have low infection potential,

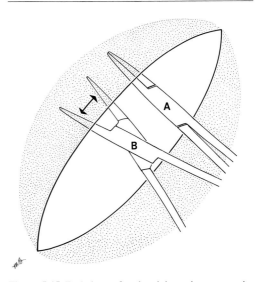

Figure 5-15 Technique of undermining using a mosquito clamp. The extent of undermining (hatched area) on both sides of the wound should roughly equal the gape of the wound. First the clamp enters to the desired depth (**A**). Next the blades are opened to bluntly dissect open the tissue plane (**B**). An iris scissors can be used also.

excellent tensile strength, and engender minimal tissue reactivity. Older materials such as silk and cotton cause greater tissue reactivity and have a higher potential for inducing infection. Hence these older materials should rarely be used (see Chapter 2).

The suture thickness needed depends on the region being repaired. For the face, use size 6-0, swaged to a small needle. For the arms, legs, feet, and trunk, use size 5-0 or 4-0. On the hands use either size 5-0 or 6-0, since larger-caliber sutures have a greater potential for ripping the skin in this region. For scalp lacerations use size 4-0 or 3-0 with large needle for a woman, but use a smaller caliber (4-0 or 5-0) for a man who has the potential for losing his hair. Prolene, which is blue in color, is easier to find in hairy regions during suture removal.

Needles. Choose a small needle for fine work, such as repairing a facial laceration. The p-3 needle is excellent for the face. For areas such as the scalp where a few large bites will suffice, choose a large cutting needle. In most cases needles are drawn to scale on the suture packages.

Suture Loop Configuration

To aid in edge eversion, the base of the suture loop should be as wide or wider than the top of the suture loop.

Avoid having the suture loop narrow at the base of the wound (as shown in Fig. 5-4A), but rather have the loop as broad at the base as at the top (as shown in Figure 5-4B). When the loop is closed by tying the stitch, the greater tissue in the lower portion of the loop will push the upper portion up creating edge eversion. If too little tissue is at the base of the loop, the edges will tend to invert.

Spacing of Sutures

The closer the suture is to the wound edge, the better the control over that edge. Hence for plastic closures, the suture should enter and exit the skin about 2 mm from the edge, and at a depth about 2 mm from the surface. In most cases the point of exit should be directly across from the point of entry. The distance between sutures should be between 2 and 6 mm, depending on the tissue. Space sutures equal distances apart along the entire extent of the laceration. For better cosmetic effect, use many small stitches set close together. On the face, for example, the sutures should be placed 2 mm from the wound edge and approximately 2 to 3 mm apart, as shown in Figure 5-16. On other parts of the body the sutures are placed farther from the wound edge and further apart.

Technique of Suture Placement

Grasp the needle with the needle holder one-third to one-half of the way down the needle from the point where the suture attaches. In this area the needles are flattened giving the needle holders a larger surface to hold onto.

Hold the needle holder in the palm, using the index finger for fine control, as shown in Figure 5-17. Many novices attempt to suture keeping the thumb and finger in the finger-holes. This can be likened to trying to write with a pencil when holding on to only the eraser end.

It is easiest to suture toward oneself, as opposed to away from oneself. Thus, enter at the far side of the wound and exit on the near side.

During suturing, control the wound edges using either a skin hook or a small forceps such as an adson forceps.

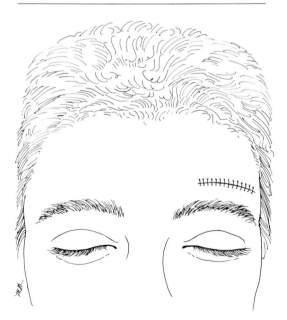

Figure 5-16 Spacing of sutures. On the face the sutures should be placed approximately 2 mm from the wound edge and 2 to 3 mm apart.

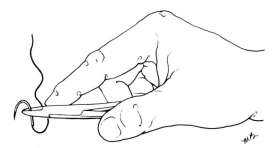

Figure 5-17 Palming the needle holder. This grasp offers better control than holding with one's fingers in the fingerholes.

Treat the tissue as gently as possible. When forceps are employed, be sure not to crush the tissue. Some authors recommend grasping only the deep tissue with the forceps, to avoid puncturing or crushing the skin itself.[45]

One of the most commonly made errors is to enter the skin with the needle tip almost parallel to the plane of the skin. If this error is made, the resulting loop will have too little tissue at the base, and consequently the edges will invert rather than evert. Rather, the needle should enter the skin at approximately a 90 degree angle. Entering at 90 degrees will increase the amount of tissue at the base of the loop (Fig. 5-18).

Axiom: One of the most common mistakes made in suturing is to enter the skin tangential instead of perpendicular to the skin plane.

The angle of entry of the needle is not as important in fine repairs in which the skin sutures are relatively shallow and placed close to the wound edge.

Uplifting the skin edge as the needle enters further increases the amount of tissue at the base of the suture loop. The edge can be uplifted either with a forceps or a skin hook. Alternatively, in some instances simply pushing down on the skin 1 cm from the wound edge will cause that edge to uplift, even without the use of a forceps or hook (Fig. 5-19).

Similarly, uplifting the opposite wound edge as the needle exits will cause there to be adequate tissue at the base of the suture loop on that side as well (Fig. 5-20A). Alternatively, one can exit the skin by coursing the needle an extra 2 to 3 mm in the deep tissue plane prior to rotating the needle out of the skin (Fig. 5-20B).

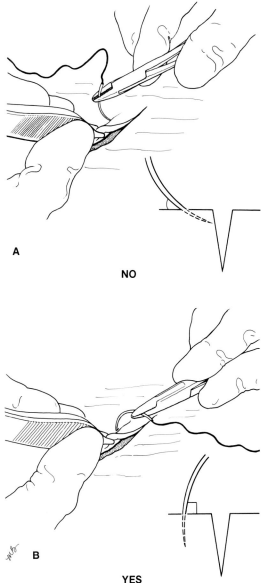

A

NO

B

YES

Figure 5-18 A. Do not enter the skin with the needle at a tangent, as this will yield too little tissue at the base of the suture loop. **B.** The skin should be entered at a 90 degree angle. See text for details.

Both technqiues are equally acceptable, but uplifting the edge is more time consuming.

For most lacerations the suture should lie at the same depth on both sides of the wound. In other words, the level at which the needle exits the tissue on one side of the wound must be the same as the level which it reenters on the other side. If these levels are different, then a ledge in the skin will form, as shown in Figure 5-21.

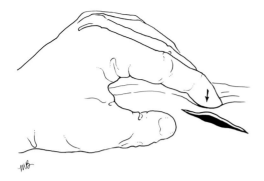

Figure 5-19 Pushing down on the skin 1 cm from the wound edge will cause that edge to lift up.

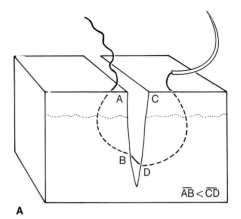

A

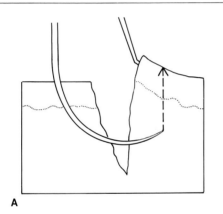

A

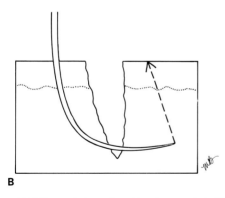

B

Figure 5-20 Two techniques for exiting the wound. **A**. The edge is uplifted as the needle exits. **B**. The needle courses an extra 2 to 3 mm in the deep tissue prior to being rotated out of the skin. The hatched line indicates the final path the needle takes.

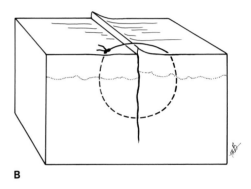

B

Figure 5-21. A and **B**. The depth of the suture must be identical on both sides of the laceration, or a ledge will occur when the suture is tied (as seen in **B**).

terials tend to unravel when improperly tied. The strands of suture material need to intertwine in alternate directions with each throw in order for the knot to square. Squaring is essential for maintaining knot security.

For nylon and Prolene, use a total of four to five throws per knot. For silk and cotton, only a total of three throws are needed.

Instrument Tie. The instrument tie is illustrated in Figure 5-22.

First, make the suture loop in the usual manner. Then hold the end of the suture that is swaged to the needle (initially, the end exiting the near side of the wound, if the suture was placed by entering far side and exiting the near side) with the nondominant hand, and pull on the suture until the free end on the other side of the wound is only about 2 to 4 cm in length. Hold the needle holder with the dominant hand. Next,

Tying the Knot

General Principles. Proper knot tying procedure must be adhered to strictly, especially when using nylon and Prolene, since these ma-

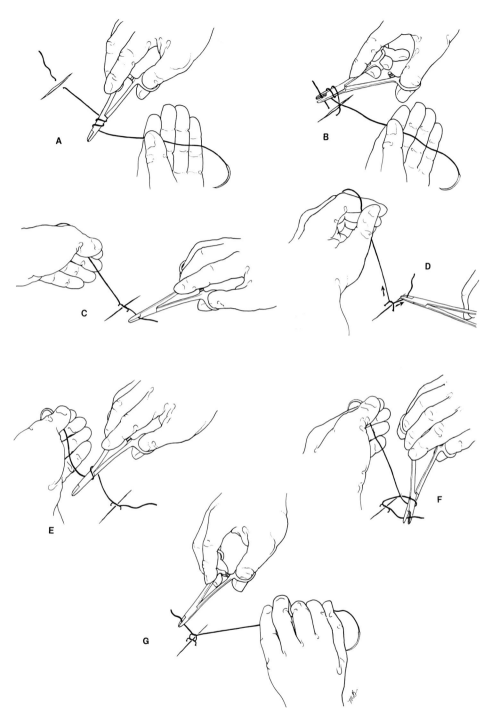

Figure 5-22 The instrument tie. During the instrument tie, manipulate the needle end of the suture with the nondominant hand and the needle holder with the dominant hand. To start with, the suture enters the far side and exits the near side of the wound in the usual fashion. **A**. Lay the needle holder on the suture on the near side, and then wrap the suture around the needle holder twice. **B**. Next reach back with the needle holders and grab the free suture end on the far side. **C**. Cross hands, pulling the free end back toward the near side and bringing the needle end of the suture to the far side. **D**. Lift up both suture ends and cinch down the first throw. **E**. Now lay the needle holder on the suture on the far side and loop once. **F**. Reach back and grab the free suture end. **G**. Cross hands and the knot will square. Repeat this pattern for a total of four to five throws.

loop the swaged end of the suture twice around the needle holder for monofilament suture materials (a single loop suffices with most braided sutures such as silk and Dexon). Then grab the free end of suture with the blades of the needle holder. After the free end of the suture is grasped, cross the hands so that the hand holding the swaged end is on the far side, and the hand holding the needle holder and the free end are on the near side of the wound. Pull upward on the suture ends when cinching the first throw of the knot. This lifting up is a simple and effective means of obtaining edge eversion.

Carefully adjust the final tension of the first throw, so that the wound edges come together snugly, but not tightly. If the loop is too tight, local tissue necrosis will occur. If it is too loose, the edges will come out of alignment.

For the second throw of the knot, the needle end is on the far side of the wound and the free end on the near side. Again, hold the needle end of the suture in the nondominant hand and lay the needle holder on top. Loop the suture only once around the needle holder, again reach back and grasp the free end within the blades of the holder, and then cross the hands so that the sutures smoothly intertwine. Take care not to cinch down too tightly on the second throw, because the tightness will be transmitted to the wound, especially if a monofilament suture material is being used. If the knotting has been properly done, the knot will square. Pull the knot to one side so that it will not directly overlie the laceration.

The pattern of looping the suture around the holder on alternate sides of the wound is repeated until there are a total of four to five throws in the final knot. The last throw can be cinched firmly, without transmitting the tension to the suture loop. For monofilaments, cut the ends long, approximately 3 to 5 mm. For most braided materials, such as silk and cotton, the ends can be cut short—2 mm.

The instrument tie has the advantage over the hand tie in that less suture material is required, but it provides less control in wounds that have high extrinsic tension.

Two-Hand Tie. The two-hand tie is illustrated in Figure 5-23. One must use special cau-

tion when using this technique in a suture with an attached needle, to avoid being punctured with the needle. The method is best suited when using free ligatures to tie off bleeding vessels.

One-Hand Tie. With the one-hand tie, one hand forms the alternating knots with the free end of the suture, while the other hand holds the swaged end secure.

Single-Layer Closure

General. The single-layer closure is the technique of choice for repairing most of the lacerations that are treated in an emergency department. It is essentially the only repair used on hands and feet, where deep sutures are shunned because of the increased potential for infection. Most lacerations of the extremities, trunk, and scalp require only one layer. The face, however, is frequently not amenable to a single-layer repair, because of the need to properly approximate the muscles of facial expression, as well as to avoid pitting in the region of the repair.

Technique. Before beginning the repair, look at the wound, decide on how far the sutures should be placed from one another, and how far from the wound edge.

As mentioned already, for facial lacerations the sutures should be 1 to 2 mm from the edge, and 2 to 3 mm apart. For other areas of the body place the sutures 2 to 4 mm from the edge, and up to 6 mm apart (the spacing of sutures is discussed further in Chapter 8).

There are basically two methods for closing a laceration: either to start at one end of the wound and work down to the other end, or to repeatedly bisect the wound until the wound is closed. Both techniques are acceptable. However, only after the technique of starting at one end and working to the other has been mastered can one proceed to learn the running suture technique discussed in Chapter 6. Some practitioners shy away from beginning at one end and working to the other end for fear that a tissue buckle (usually referred to as a ''dog-ear'') will appear toward the end of the repair. However, by making small adjustments in the amount of tissue taken on each side of the wound with each stitch with each suture, dog ear deformities can be avoided.

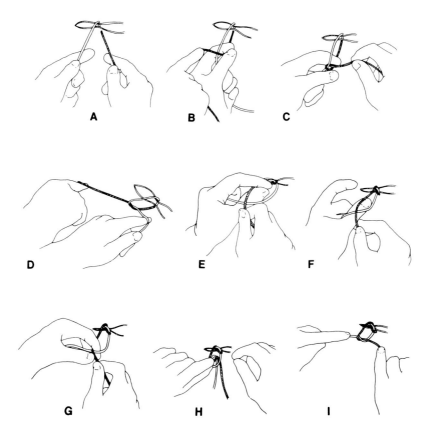

Figure 5-23 The two-hand tie. *Source:* Reprinted from *Minor Injuries and Disorders: Surgical and Medical Care* (p 62) by J Grossman with permission of JB Lippincott Company, © 1984.

For example, often the two sides of a wound are of different lengths, most often due to differential stress on the skin on the two sides. Normally the points of entry and exit are directly across from one another. However, in this case, space the sutures farther apart on the longer side than the shorter side of the wound (Fig. 5-24).

When there are definite landmarks, such as the eyebrow, vermilion border of the lip, or the deep creases in the palm, place the first suture so as to bring the landmark into alignment. The remaining laceration on either side of the landmark is then repaired in the usual fashion.

The Simple Deep Suture

General

As already mentioned, repair of the deep layers of a laceration improves the final, cosmetic appearance of the repair. For most deep repairs the authors recommend either Vycril or Dexon, which are both stronger and less pyogenic than natural materials such as chromic and plain gut (see Chapter 2).

Unlike skin sutures, where placing sutures relatively close together improves the repair, with deep sutures use the minimum number of ties that will bring the tissues securely together, since suture marks will not be a problem. However, bear in mind that the more foreign material within the wound, the greater the risk of infection.

Deep sutures must be placed in collagen-containing tissues. The fatty or muscular layer alone will not hold the suture.

Deep sutures are to be avoided in the distal extremities, where the risk of infection and the risk of inadvertently catching a tendon or nerve

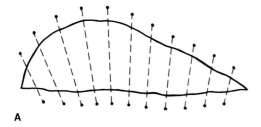

A

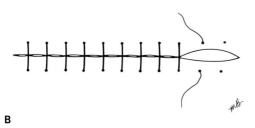

B

Figure 5-24 Repairing lacerations in which the two sides are of different lengths. **A**. The far side of the wound is of greater length than the near side, owing to different amounts of stress on the tissues. The sutures are not placed directly across the wound from one another as is usually the case, but are spaced in such a manner as to accommodate the extra length of the far side. **B**. The wound closes without buckling.

within the deep suture loop are both high. As a rule, no deep sutures should be placed in the hand.

Buried Knot Suture

For the emergency department repair of lacerations, the most useful deep stitch is the simple buried knot suture (Fig. 5-25). The loop is constructed so that the knot lies at the bottom, leaving the upper surface that the skin will rest on smooth and flat. The needle enters the deep portion of the tissue to be repaired first, and exits at a more superficial plane. Next the needle enters the opposite side of the wound at the same superficial plane and exits at the deep plane.

It is usually easiest to tie the knot from one side, rather than from directly above the suture loop. As with skin sutures, the edges should be carefully approximated, but not cinched down under undue tension. Since Vycril and Dexon are braided, the first throw can be a single as opposed to a double loop, only a total of three

throws are needed, and the ends can be cut short. After the knot is tied and the sutures cut, use a closed needle holder or other instrument to push the knot to its proper position at the base of the wound.

A common mistake which is quite easy to make is to allow one strand of the suture to overlie the top of the loop prior to tying the knot,

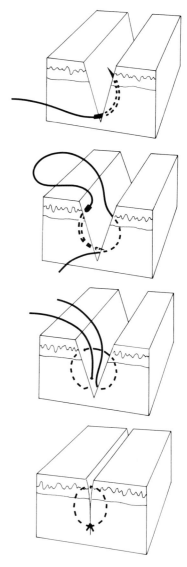

Figure 5-25 The buried knot suture. See text for discussion. *Source:* Reprinted from *Procedures and Techniques in Emergency Medicine* (p 295) by RR Simon and BE Brenner with permission of the Williams & Wilkins Company, Baltimore, © 1982.

as illustrated in Figure 5-26. Thus, the physician should take care that neither strand overlies the top of the loop prior to knotting.

In some cases the deep sutures along a wound must all be placed prior to tying each knot, because the tying of one suture can make the placement of the subsequent deep sutures more difficult. Once all sutures are in place, the knots can be tied.

After the deep repair is complete, run a finger along the repaired layer. If there are valleys or ruts for the finger to fall into, then additional deep sutures are needed.

Some wounds require repairs to more than two layers (i.e., deep and skin). For example, if a deep muscle is lacerated, the muscle sheath should be repaired, followed by the subcutaneous tissue, and then the skin. In cases of injuries to multiple deep layers, only the most superficial layer need be constructed with the knot buried at the bottom of the suture loop. The other sutures can be tied in the standard method with the knot on top.

Other Adjuncts to Skin Closure

Skin Tape (See also Chapter 2)

General. Skin tapes, when properly used, can yield an excellent cosmetic result. Tapes have several advantages over sutures. The wound infection rates are lower. There is no potential for suture mark formation. Tapes are easier to use.

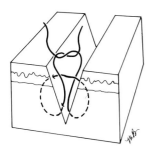

Figure 5-26 Error in buried knot suture. In this illustration, one strand of suture passes over the top of the loop and the other strand beneath. Both strands must lie beneath the loop, otherwise the knot cannot be buried.

There are many instances, however, when skin tapes are not practical. For example, tapes cannot be placed until there is total hemostasis; they will not bind to a moist field. If there is excessive sweating in the region of the wound following placement, the tapes tend to come loose. Young children tend to pull off the strips of tape prematurely. Tapes are impractical in regions of motion, such as the fingers, wrist, and elbow. Lastly, at times wound edges invert following tape placement.

Hence, tapes are useful in adults or cooperative children in regions of the body where there is not excessive motion or moisture, and where the skin edges do not invert. Small lacerations of the forehead and cheeks, for example, often heal remarkably well with skin tapes. Further, skin tape is useful for closure of wounds that are on the borderline of being too old to close, because of the decreased pyogenicity of tape. Also, skin tapes are a useful means of stabilizing a wound following suture removal, as well as stabilizing a wound closed by absorbable subcuticular sutures.

Technique. The initial preparation of the wound is as for suturing. Following preparation, the surface to be taped must be completely dry. Pressure with a sterile gauze for 10 minutes is usually adequate for stopping venous bleeding. The skin adjacent to the laceration is painted with benzoin or other adhesive. The skin tapes are then placed one at a time. The smaller the width of the tape, the greater the control of the wound edge. Place the tape first on one side of the laceration, approximate the edges, then secure the tape to the other side. Leave a space of approximately 2 mm between the strips.

After the strips have been placed, carefully inspect the wound. If there is any seepage of blood, apply direct pressure over the site for 10 minutes, repeating this maneuver if necessary. Look at the wound edges. If the edges are inverted, the strips will have to be replaced with sutures. Hence it is always a good idea to warn patients ahead of time that skin tapes may not work, and the wound might need suturing.

Skin Staples

General. Like skin tape, staples offer the advantages of rapid skin closure, a lower infection rate compared with sutures, as well as a lower potential for causing skin marks. Staples, however, afford less control of the wound edge than sutures. In addition, staples are frequently unavailable in emergency departments.

Technique. The wound is prepared in the usual fashion. Preferably deep layers are closed with absorbable sutures. The skin stapler is then used to close the skin. The exact technique used varies slightly according to the type of stapler employed.

Skin Adhesives

General. Skin adhesives are chemicals that bind to skin, allowing tissue closure in the same manner as one would glue together two pieces of wood or plastic. As with tape, the field must be completely dry. The use of adhesives has been relatively limited in the United States. Skin adhesives are rarely available in emergency departments in this country.

Technique. The adhesive is applied to both edges and allowed to set for 30 seconds. The edges are then approximated and held secure for an additional 3 minutes.

Chapter 6

Advanced Suturing Techniques

In this chapter, we will present a variety of suturing techniques, along with their indications and possible disadvantages. In practice, it is better to learn a few of these techniques well, rather than to gain a passing knowledge of all of them. For example, mastery of the simple skin suture, the deep buried knot suture, the vertical and horizontal mattresses, and the half-buried horizontal mattress stitch allows the physician to expertly repair the majority of complex lacerations that present to the emergency department.

The end of the chapter presents various specialized knotting techniques.

ADVANCED SUTURING TECHNIQUES

Simple Running Suture—Common Technique

Description (Fig. 6-1)

A *running suture* is similar to a simple suture in technique, except that the suture material is not cut and tied with each succeeding stitch. Rather, one makes and ties the first loop the same way as a simple suture, except that the suture attached to the needle is not cut. Multiple loops are then made, starting at one end of the laceration and working toward the other. For the final loop, enter the skin just beside the entry point of the preceding stitch. After all the loops are in place, adjust the tension all along the repair, being certain that none of the stitches are too tight. Finally, complete the repair by tying the suture to itself.

Indications

The primary benefit of the running skin suture is speed. Once the technique has been mastered, the final cosmetic appearance of the scar is comparable to interrupted skin sutures. The running suture is easier to remove since fewer loops need to be cut. Therefore the technique is particularly attractive for use with uncooperative young children, as well as in cases where multiple small sutures are placed.

Disadvantages

The main drawback of the running suture is that if the suture breaks anywhere along the repair, the whole suture line can unravel. In addition, if a mistake is made placing a suture loop, the suture must be cut, the loop removed, and a knot placed at the previous loop. The running repair must then be reinitiated. There is therefore generally a greater tendency to leave in place an imperfect loop with the running technique than with the interrupted technique.

Simple Running Suture—Alternate Method with Suture Perpendicular to the Laceration Line

Description

In the normal *simple running skin closure*, the suture runs at a diagonal to the wound edge on the surface and at a perpendicular angle below the surface, as shown in Figure 6-1. A slight modification reverses this pattern, causing the suture to be aligned perpendicular to the wound edge on the surface and at a diagonal below the skin.

Again, the repair is begun similarly to a simple skin suture, but without cutting the suture end that is attached to the needle. The knot is then pulled to the side of the wound where the skin was initially entered. Next the skin is reentered immediately adjacent to the knot, and the needle is made to track beneath the surface of the skin at approximately a 60-degree angle, as shown in Figure 6-2. On the surface, run the suture at a perpendicular to the wound edge. In making the final loop, course the needle beneath the skin so the suture exits just adjacent to the exit point of the previous loop. Then the repair is completed by securing the suture to itself, as in the standard technique.

Indications and Disadvantages

The indications and drawbacks for this technique are the same as for the regular running suture. Some practitioners prefer the perpendicular pattern of sutures of the alternate technique. The alternate technique is harder to master. Neither variety of continuous suture has advantage over the other in terms of the final appearance of the laceration.

Locked Running Suture

Description

The *locked running suture* is similar to the simple running suture, except that the suture is

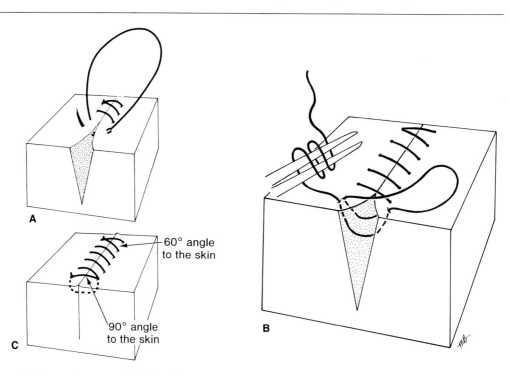

Figure 6-1 The running suture. **A.** Begin with a simple suture at one end of the wound, and then run down the length of the laceration. **B** and **C.** To complete the repair, knot the suture to itself. By using this technique the suture lies diagonally above the skin. *Source:* Figures 6-1A and C are reprinted from *Procedures and Techniques in Emergency Medicine* (p 289) by RR Simon and BE Brenner with permission of the Williams & Wilkins Company, Baltimore, © 1982.

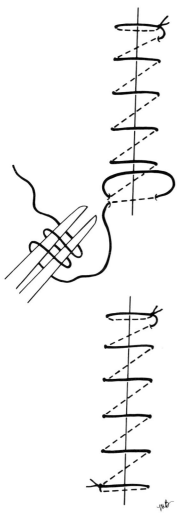

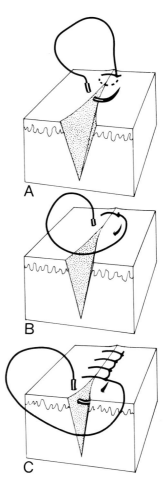

Figure 6-2 The running suture, alternate method. Note that the suture runs perpendicular to the wound edge on the surface (solid lines), but diagonally beneath the surface (hatched lines).

Figure 6-3 The locked running suture. **A.** The stitch is begun the same way as for a conventional running suture. **B** and **C.** The needle is then looped through the preceding surface suture. *Source:* Reprinted from *Procedures and Techniques in Emergency Medicine* (p 290) by RR Simon and BE Brenner with permission of the Williams & Wilkins Company, Baltimore, © 1982.

made to pass through the preceding loop prior to reentering the skin, as shown in Figure 6-3.

With this technique, the suture lies perpendicular to the wound edge both above and below the skin surface.

Indications

At times with the simple running suture the preceding loops loosen while the next stitch is being placed. Locking the sutures secures these preceding loops.

The locked running suture is also useful in the rare situation where the wound edges have to be pulled together under tension to control bleeding. An example is a highly vascular region such as the scalp.

Disadvantages

Some textbooks of wound repair state that the locked running suture should not be used because it is a strangulating stitch. Any technique strangulates the tissues if the sutures are cinched down too tightly. If the physician takes care to approximate with appropriate tension, tissue strangulation will not be a problem.

The locked technique takes slightly more time to execute than the simple running technique but this difference becomes negligible with practice.

Vertical Mattress Suture

Description

The *mattress technique* involves placing a double line of suture material across the wound. The skin is entered and exited twice, instead of only once as occurs with simple sutures. Simple sutures, by comparison, have only a single strand of suture inside the tissues.

With a vertical mattress suture, the two lines of suture lie one above the other. The technique is begun in the same way as a simple skin suture, but the wound is entered and exited a generous distance from the edge. Then the needle is resecured to the holder and with a backhand technique the wound is reentered and exited about 1 to 2 mm from the edge. The suture is tied in the usual fashion (Fig. 6-4).

Indications

The vertical mattress technique insures wound edge eversion. Thus the technique is especially useful in areas of the body where the wound edges have a tendency to invert, such as the dorsum of the hand and the volar surface of the wrist.

The physician can repair the entire laceration with vertical mattress stitches, or alternate mattress ties with simple ties.

Disadvantages

Each vertical mattress suture loop requires four points of skin entry and exit as compared to two for a simple suture and hence is more time consuming. Also, if suture track marks occur, there are twice as many as with simple sutures.

Horizontal Mattress Suture—
Standard Method

Description

With a *horizontal mattress suture,* the two lines of suture lie parallel to one another in a

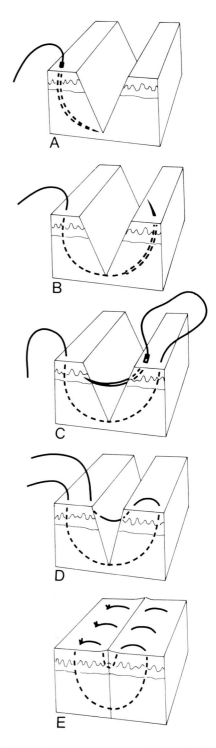

Figure 6-4 The vertical mattress suture. See text for discussion. *Source:* Reprinted from *Procedures and Techniques in Emergency Medicine* (p 291) by RR Simon and BE Brenner with permission of the Williams & Wilkins Company, Baltimore, © 1982.

horizontal plane, as shown in Figure 6-5. First, the needle enters on the far side of the wound and exits on the near side as in a standard simple suture. The pattern is then reversed, with the needle entering on the near side and exiting on the far side. The suture is then tied in the usual fashion.

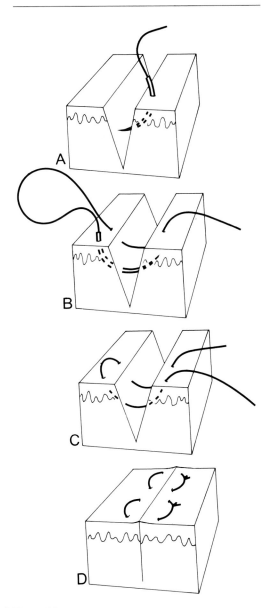

Figure 6-5 The horizontal mattress stitch. See text for discussion. *Source:* Reprinted from *Procedures and Techniques in Emergency Medicine* (p 292) by RR Simon and BE Brenner with permission of the Williams & Wilkins Company, Baltimore, © 1982.

Indications

First, because the suture tension is exerted from either side of the wound (as opposed to over the top of the wound as with a simple tie), the horizontal mattress suture everts the skin edge even more powerfully than the vertical mattress suture. Hence, this stitch, too, is useful in areas where edge inversion is a problem.

Second, a single horizontal mattress stitch can take the place of two simple ties to repair a small laceration, thus saving time.

Third, the horizontal mattress sutures are less likely to rip through the skin, and therefore the technique is useful in areas where the skin is atrophic, such as the lower leg in elderly patients.

Disadvantages

If the horizontal mattress suture is secured under undue tension, the suture will pucker the tissue within the loop. This stitch also affords less control of the wound edge than either the simple suture or the vertical mattress suture.

Horizontal Mattress Suture—Modified Method

As noted above, one of the main disadvantages of the standard horizontal mattress suture is poor wound edge control. By keeping the entry and exit points of each mattress stitch close together, greater wound edge control can be obtained, as shown in Figure 6-6.

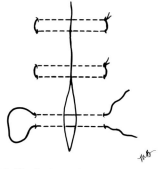

Figure 6-6 The horizontal mattress suture, modified method. Note that the entry and exit points of the suture are more closely spaced than with the conventional horizontal mattress suture.

Running Horizontal Mattress Suture

As with a simple suture, the horizontal mattress suture can be run across the length of a laceration, as illustrated in Figure 6-7.

Inverting Horizontal Mattress Suture

The term ''horizontal mattress suture'' generally refers to the everting stitch described above.

The *inverting horizontal mattress suture* is performed in a similar manner. To execute this stitch, a loop parallel to the edge is made first on the near side, and then on the far side of the wound, and the suture is tied in the usual manner (Fig. 6-8). The degree of edge inversion is determined by the degree of tension with which the knot is cinched down.

This stitch is actually rarely indicated in emergency department wound repair. Since inversion of the skin edges delays wound healing, the inverting horizontal mattress suture should not be used for skin closure but only for repairing deep tissues. Its main use is to create a smooth, inverted suture line when repairing a lacerated muscle sheath that is just beneath the skin, such as on the forearm.

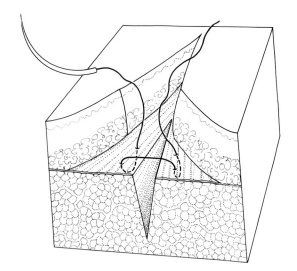

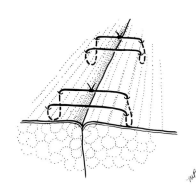

Figure 6-8 The inverting horizontal mattress suture. Unlike the conventional horizontal mattress suture, this stitch causes the wound edges to invert.

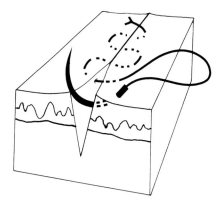

Figure 6-7 The running horizontal mattress suture. The technique is the same as for a conventional horizontal mattress suture, except that the suture is not cut and tied with each stitch. *Source:* Reprinted from *Procedures and Techniques in Emergency Medicine* (p 294) by RR Simon and BE Brenner with permission of the Williams & Wilkins Company, Baltimore, © 1987.

Half-Buried Horizontal Mattress Suture

Description

In the *half-buried horizontal mattress stitch,* as the name implies, half of the loop is above the skin and the other half below. The needle enters the skin on one side of the wound and exits at the subcuticular level of the wound edge, that is, just below the dermal-epidermal junction. Next, the physician makes a loop in the opposite wound edge, keeping the suture entirely within the subcuticular plane and insuring that it never exits to the surface on that side. The original wound edge is then reentered in the subcuticular plane and the suture is brought out directly across from the original entry point (Fig. 6-9).

The levels of entry and exit of the buried portion of the suture must be at the same depth at all points or a ledge will form.

Indications

By keeping within the subcuticular plane, use of the half-buried horizontal mattress suture avoids the vascular compromise that often occurs when small tissue flaps are repaired with a simple skin suture. It should be kept in mind that the nutrient blood vessels in the skin lie within the dermis. When the physician keeps suturing at the level of the dermal-epidermal junction, the nutrient blood vessels are not compromised.

The half-buried horizontal mattress suture is without equal in allowing for closure of complex wounds with multiple flaps. In a T-shaped wound, for example, this suture allows the closure of the region where the three wound edges meet. The skin is entered on the most intact surface, then the two flap edges are secured in the subcuticular plane, and finally the skin is exited directly across from the initial point of entry, as shown in Figure 6-10D.

The technique can also be used to bring together the multiple edges of a stellate laceration (see Fig. 6-10A–C).

The physician using the half-buried horizontal mattress suture should first locate the most intact portion of the wound, where the various edges intersect. The most intact surface is the point of entry and exit of the suture, and also the region

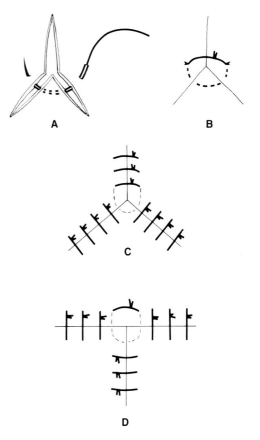

Figure 6-10 Various applications of the half-buried horizontal mattress suture. **A, B,** and **C.** Repair of a stellate laceration. **D.** The suture is used to repair a T-shaped laceration. *Source:* Reprinted from *Procedures and Techniques in Emergency Medicine* (p 293) by RR Simon and BE Brenner with permission of the Williams & Wilkins Company, Baltimore, © 1982.

of the final knot. The various wound edges are then secured in the deep plane. Fine nonabsorbable suture, such as 6-0 nylon, should be used.

The half-buried horizontal mattress suture is the method of choice for closing complex portions of wounds in parts of the body where elliptical excisions are not practical, such as the nose, ear, and face.

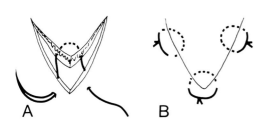

Figure 6-9 The half-buried horizontal mattress suture. Half of the suture lies beneath the skin, in the subcuticular plane (dashed lines). *Source:* Reprinted from *Procedures and Techniques in Emergency Medicine* (p 293) by RR Simon and BE Brenner with permission of the Williams & Wilkins Company, Baltimore, © 1982.

Disadvantages

If the suture is not properly placed on the first or second attempt, a third attempt is often impossible because of maceration of the subcuticular tissue of the skin flaps.

The Subcuticular Suture

Description

The subcuticular stitch is essentially a running horizontal mattress stitch that is placed just below the dermal-epidermal junction.

There are several methods of initiating the subcuticular stitch. Probably the easiest is to enter the skin 3 to 4 mm from one end of the laceration, and then burrow through the deep tissue to emerge in the subcuticular plane at the apex of the wound, as shown in Figure 6-11. Next, the suture is made to pass through the subcuticular tissue on alternate sides of the wound. The point of entry of each stitch should be directly across from, or slightly behind the exit point of the previous stitch.

Be certain to be gentle when handling the tissue, since there is a tendency to bear down too hard with forceps when working in the subcuticular region.

When the repair is completed, the needle again burrows through the dermis, and is made to exit the skin. Prior to securing the suture ends in place, the tension along the wound should be carefully adjusted to insure that there is no puckering of the skin.

The free suture at both ends of the laceration can then be taped into place, as shown in Figure 6-11.

Suture material for the subcuticular stitch should be of narrow caliber, either 5-0 or 6-0. If a nonabsorbable material is employed, then the stitch should be stopped and restarted every 3 to 4 cm to facilitate subsequent suture removal.

The authors recommend placing a layer of steri-strips or other skin tapes over the repaired region to add additional support after the suture is removed. Skin tapes are not needed if an absorbable material such as Vycril or Dexon is used, since these materials take several weeks to absorb.

Indications

Placing sutures in the subcuticular region avoids the problem of suture marks, while at the same time allowing for excellent skin edge eversion. The repair is best suited to straight lacerations.

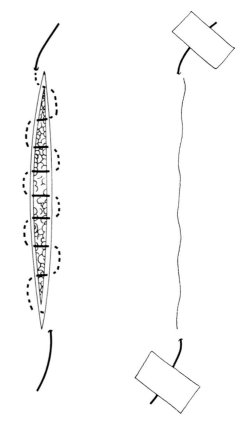

Figure 6-11 The subcuticular suture. See text for discussion. *Source:* Reprinted from *Procedures and Techniques in Emergency Medicine* (p 294) by RR Simon and BE Brenner with permission of the Williams & Wilkins Company, Baltimore, © 1982.

This closure with an absorbable suture material is excellent in cases where the patient cannot be relied on to return for suture removal.

Disadvantages

The technique is harder to learn and takes more time to perform than simple, running percutaneous sutures. In one study of pediatric patients undergoing elective surgery, there was no significant difference in the cosmetic appearance of wounds repaired with subcuticular as compared to percutaneous sutures.[65]

Buried Horizontal Mattress Suture

Description

As an alternative to the simple buried suture described in Chapter 5, deep tissues can be closed with a buried horizontal mattress stitch. Parallel bites of tissues are taken from both sides of the wound and the suture is tied, as illustrated in Figure 6-12.

Indications

There are two main indications for the buried horizontal mattress stitch. First, a single buried horizontal mattress often can take the place of two, separate buried simple sutures. Hence the deep layer can be repaired more rapidly, and with less buried suture material. Second, the buried horizontal mattress is easier to place in shallow wounds that require a layered closure, such as on the face.

Disadvantages

If the entry and exit points on both sides are not at identical depths, a ledge will form at the surface of the wound. If the bites of tissue taken from either side of the wound are not equal in size, a pucker will result. If the bites taken are too large, a dimple in the skin will occur adjacent to the repair.

Reinforced Suture

Description

Sterile cotton pledgets or sterile buttons are placed at the entry and exit points of a conven-

tional horizontal mattress suture, thus increasing the area of skin that supports the closure (Fig. 6-13).

Indications

This technique is particularly useful in patients with thin, easily damaged skin. The most common instances are elderly patients and patients on corticosteroids.

Disadvantages

Essentially none.

Retention Sutures

Description

Retention sutures are broad, deep skin stitches that enter and exit the skin at an increased distance from the wound edge. Placing a few retension sutures along a laceration decreases the

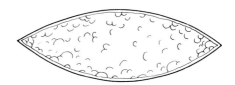

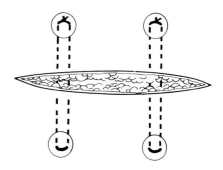

Figure 6-13 The reinforced suture. Sterile cotton pledgets or sterile buttons can be used to reinforce a horizontal mattress suture. *Source:* Reprinted from *Procedures and Techniques in Emergency Medicine* (p 297) by RR Simon and BE Brenner with permission of the Williams & Wilkins Company, Baltimore, © 1982.

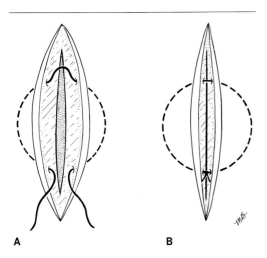

A   **B**

Figure 6-12 The buried horizontal mattress suture. See text for discussion.

tension at the wound edge, as shown in Figure 6-14.

Because the tissue near the wound edge can be weakened by the normal activity of wound collagenase, the retention sutures should be at least 6 to 7 mm from the wound edge.[104]

A strong suture should be used, such as 2-0 nylon or steel.

Indications

This technique is most frequently used in the closure of abdominal operative wounds and is rarely used in emergency medicine. One indication would be to reinforce the skin sutures in a patient with atrophic skin.

Disadvantages

The main disadvantage is additional foreign material in the wound, and the potential for added suture marks.

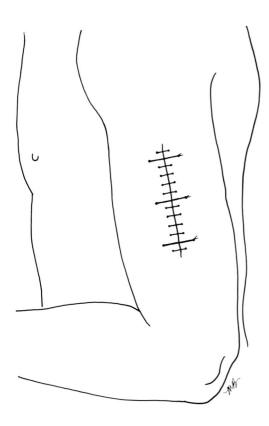

Figure 6-14 Retention sutures. See text for discussion.

ADVANCED KNOTTING TECHNIQUES

Slip Knot

Description

The *slip knot* is made by keeping a loop in the free end of the suture during tying, as shown in Figure 6-15.

Pulling on the free end unravels the knot.

Indications

The slip knot facilitates suture removal, which is often difficult in pediatric patients.

Disadvantages

With the newer suture materials, such as nylon and polypropylene, knot security is a problem even with standard knotting techniques. Therefore the slip knot, which has even less knot security, is not particularly practical, despite its advantage of easy removal.

Open Loop Knot

Description

With this knot, a loop is maintained between the first and second throws of the knot. Normally, this loop is obliterated when one cinches down the knot after the second throw. Hence, by not cinching down all the way, a small loop is maintained (Fig. 6-16).

Indications

This technique is especially useful with suture materials with a high degree of ''memory'' (i.e., those that do not lie flat during suturing), such as nylon and polypropylene. These materials have a tendency to contort the wound edges when the second throw is cinched down fully, especially in regions such as the eyelid where the skin is extremely thin. With the open loop knot the distortion does not occur.

The technique allows for edema. Thus it is useful in instances where edema is expected, such as compression injuries.

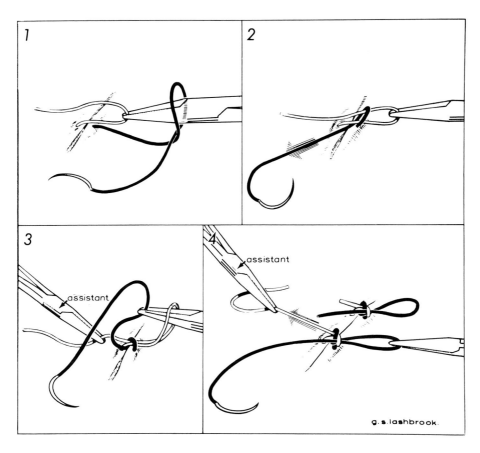

Figure 6-15 The slip-knot. *Source:* Reprinted with permission from "The Interlocking Slip Knot" by ML Lucid, *Plastic and Reconstructive Surgery* (1964;34:200), Copyright © 1964, Williams & Wilkins Company, Baltimore.

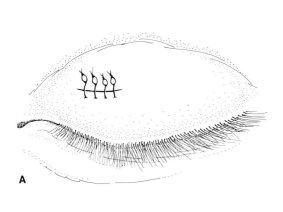

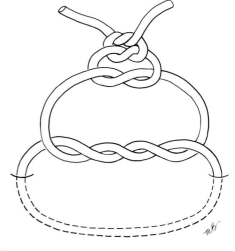

Figure 6-16 The open loop knot. The second throw is not cinched down all the way, leaving a small loop.

Disadvantages

If the open loop knot is made too large, appropriate skin tension may be lost, causing the wound to gape.

Two-Instrument Tie

Description

The knot is tied similar to a classic instrument tie, except that constant tension is held on the free end with a second instrument (Fig. 6-17).

Indications

This technique is useful when the first throw loosens prior to cinching the second throw, such as occurs with gaping scalp lacerations. In many instances, however, the tendency of the first throw to loosen is a sign that tissues have not been adequately undermined.

Disadvantages

None.

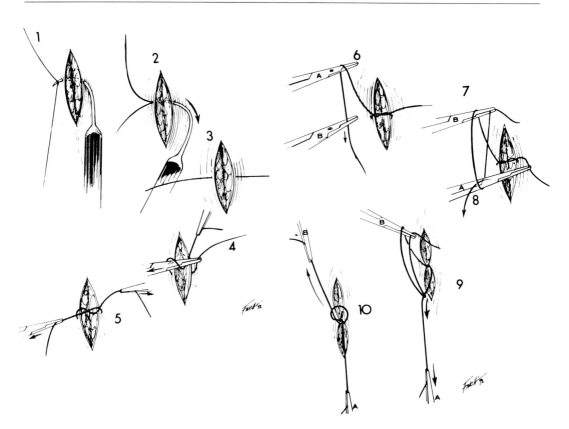

Figure 6-17 Two-instrument tie. *Source:* Reprinted with permission from *Surgery, Gynecology & Obstetrics* (1973;137:669), Copyright © 1973, Franklin H Martin Memorial Foundation.

Chapter 7

Special Techniques for Complicated Wounds

This chapter deals with a variety of techniques useful in repairing more complicated wounds such as complex lacerations, tissue defects, contaminated wounds, and flap lacerations. The techniques discussed include advancement flaps, "dog ear" repair, delayed primary closure, skin grafting, and Z-plasty. The chapter is organized by wound type and configuration, instead of by specific procedures, to facilitate being able to find the proper means of repairing a specific wound.

CLOSING A DEFECT

General

There are two causes of skin defects in lacerations. The first is simply from the extrinsic tension pulling the wound edges apart. Although the defects at times appear large, there is no actual tissue loss. The second cause is the actual avulsion of skin.

Almost all defects that are not associated with actual tissue loss can be closed by using a layered repair with adequate undermining. However, in cases of actual tissue loss, the special techniques described below may be needed.

Following undermining and primary suture closure, remaining tissue defects less than the size of a dime in diameter can be left to heal in by granulation and wound contration. Larger defects require grafting or skin flaps.

Surgically produced circular and square defects often result following the elective excision of skin because of skin cancer or for other reasons. The accidental avulsion of a full-thickness circle or square of skin is relatively uncommon. Therefore, plastic surgeons and dermatologists tend to perform the more complex advancement and rotational flaps described below more often than emergency department physicians. These flaps tend to be time consuming, and in even the best hands flap necrosis can ensue. Therefore, the emergency physician should consider referring patients requiring a complex flap repair to the plastic surgeon.

Elliptical Defects

General

Lacerations generally take on an elliptical configuration due to extrinsic tension. Most elliptical defects do not involve actual tissue loss and can be repaired using a simple or layered closure following undermining of the edges. Defects due to tissue loss, however, require special techniques for closure.

Wide ellipses most commonly result from the débridement of large, irregular lacerations. In addition, wide defects can occur without tissue loss in wounds under accentuated external tension, such as lacerations of the lower extremity in obese patients.

Closure Techniques

V-Y Advancement (Fig. 7-1). In this technique, a V-shaped incision is made on one side of the ellipse. The tissue near the V is then undermined. The result is that the skin above the ellipse is freer to advance forward, allowing for closure of the ellipse. Finally, the V itself is closed by converting the V to a Y.

The V-Y advancement is especially useful in closing small defects, such as can occur following scraping injuries over the knuckles.

The main disadvantage of the technique, as with many other flaps, is that a second defect is created and the physician must be certain there is enough mobile tissue to close the second defect.

Interpolation Flap. In the interpolation flap, a tongue-shaped flap of tissue immediately adjacent to the ellipse is transferred over to cover the ellipse. The defect created by the removal of the flap is then closed with simple sutures (Fig. 7-2).

Note that the tongue-shaped flap is narrower than the defect it is to fill, the elasticity of the tissue making up for the size differences. This technique requires that the tissue be fairly loose. Also, since the undersurface of the flap is freed from the deep tissue, the region must be well perfused. The base of the flap must be proximal to enhance perfusion.

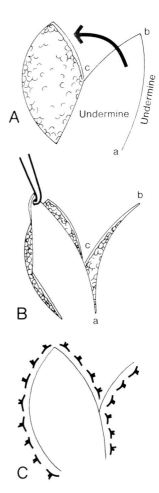

Figure 7-2 Interpolation flap, useful in closing elliptical defects. See text for discussion. *Source:* Reprinted from *Procedures and Techniques in Emergency Medicine* (p 302) by RR Simon and BE Brenner with permission of the Williams & Wilkins Company, Baltimore, © 1982.

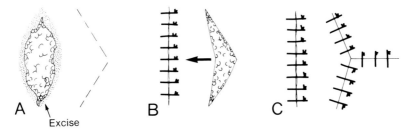

Figure 7-1 V-Y advancement for closure of an elliptical defect. **(A).** The hatched lines indicate the place to make a V-shaped incision through the skin. The original ellipse is repaired **(B)** and the secondary defect closed **(C)**. *Source:* Reprinted from *Procedures and Techniques in Emergency Medicine* (p 301) by RR Simon and BE Brenner with permission of the Williams & Wilkins Company, Baltimore, © 1982.

Circular Defects

General

Circular defects most commonly occur from excisional biopsies and other minor surgical procedures. Circular defects can occur as the result of accidental trauma, as well, however.

Closure Techniques

Conversion to An Ellipse. The easiest way to repair a circular defect is to convert the circle into an ellipse and then close, leaving a linear scar, as illustrated in Figure 7-3. The ellipse should be constructed so that the final scar is parallel to the normal skin tension lines.

The drawback of this technique is that the final linear scar is more than twice as long as the diameter of the original circle.

Sliding Triangular Pedicle Flaps.[183] When conversion of the circular defect to an ellipse necessitates excision of an unacceptable amount of skin, triangular pedicles can be advanced from opposite sides of the circle to close the defect, as shown in Figure 7-4.

The blood supply to the triangles is from the subcutaneous tissue. Therefore the tissue under the flaps must be left intact. The technique is only practical in areas with excellent perfusion, such as the face.

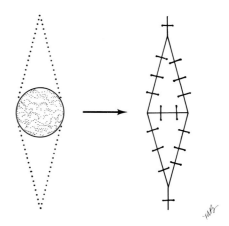

Figure 7-4 Triangular advancement flap closure of a circular defect. Two triangles of tissue are formed by incising the skin along the dotted lines in the drawing on the left. The flaps then slide forward to close the circle, as shown in the illustration on the right. The tissue under the flaps must be left intact, otherwise the flaps will necrose.

Triangular Defects

General

Triangular defects often follow tangential lacerations in which a slice of tissue is avulsed off.

Closure Techniques

Conversion to an Ellipse. First, undermine. This will make the size of the triangle smaller by freeing up the edges. Next, excise a mirror image of tissue from the base to convert the triangle into an ellipse. The ellipse is then closed in the usual fashion (Fig. 7-5).

Rotation Flap. With the *rotation flap*, tissue adjacent to the triangle is incised in a semicircular fashion to allow closure of the triangle, as shown in Figure 7-6. The subcutaneous tissue of the flap is undermined. The drawback is that a large, arcuate laceration is created alongside the original defect.

Square or Rectangular Defects

General

A variety of mechanisms of injuries, including motor vehicle accidents, can cause tissue

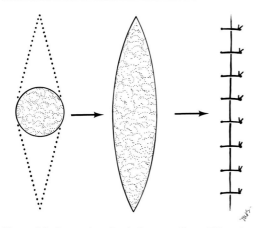

Figure 7-3 Conversion of a circle to an ellipse. This technique allows for closure of the circle without the formation of buckles in the neighboring skin. The dotted lines in the illustration on the left indicate the pattern of excision. The drawing on the right shows the finished repair.

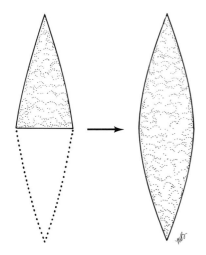

Figure 7-5 Conversion of a triangle to an ellipse. This method is most useful when the base of the triangle is narrow.

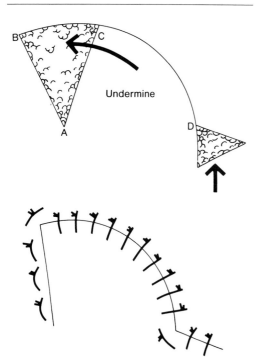

Figure 7-6 Closure of a triangular defect with a rotation flap. The original defect is triangle ABC. A small wedge is excised at point D, to avoid skin buckling when the flap is rotated. In the lower illustration the flap has been rotated into place. The half-buried horizontal mattress stitch is employed to suture close the left-hand side of the wound, and the small corner on the right, to decrease the risk of ischemia. *Source:* Reprinted from *Procedures and Techniques in Emergency Medicine* (p 301) by RR Simon and BE Brenner with permission of the Williams & Wilkins Company, Baltimore, © 1982.

avulsions that leave square or rectangular defects. Fortunately, most of the time the defects are small.

Closure Techniques

Conversion to an Ellipse. As with the other defects described already, conversion to an ellipse is the simplest technique of repair, especially for narrow rectangular wounds, as shown in Figure 7-7.

Advancement flap.[86] A simple rectangular advancement flap can be used to close both rectangular and square defects. The length/width ratio should not exceed 2:1. Be sure that the base of the flap is proximal, to enhance perfusion. Undermining of the flap should be kept to a minimum. Small wedges of tissue often need to be excised from the base of the flap to avoid bunching-up of the tissue (Fig. 7-8).

Diamond-shaped (Rhomboid) Defects[81]

Conversion to an Ellipse

As with other defects, a diamond-shaped lesion, especially of narrow width, can be converted into an ellipse and then closed.

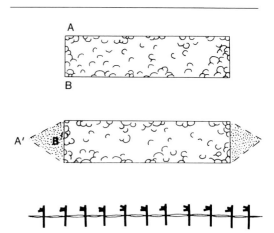

Figure 7-7 Conversion of a rectangular defect into an ellipse. The height of the triangle (A' B') equals the width of the rectangle (AB). *Source:* Reprinted from *Procedures and Techniques in Emergency Medicine* (p 301) by RR Simon and BE Brenner with permission of the Williams & Wilkins Company, Baltimore, © 1982.

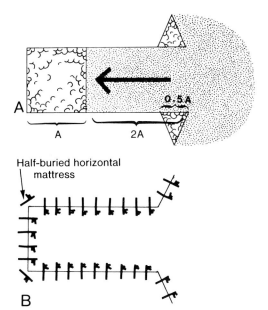

Figure 7-8 Closure of a square defect using an advancement flap. See text for discussion. *Source:* Reprinted from *Procedures and Techniques in Emergency Medicine* (p 299) by RR Simon and BE Brenner with permission of the Williams & Wilkins Company, Baltimore, © 1982.

Transposition Flap (Limberg Flap)

The *transposition flap* to close a diamond-shaped defect is essentially the same as the closure technique described above for large elliptical lesions (Fig. 7-9). The base of the flap should be proximal, to maximize perfusion.

Extensive Tissue Loss

General

The techniques listed for the closure of various-shaped defects can be applied only to relatively small lesions in well-perfused regions of the body such as the face. A wound with more extensive tissue, or in an area that is not well perfused, should be repaired with a skin graft.

Skin grafts can be either partial thickness or full thickness. Split-thickness grafts consist of primarily the epidermis, while full-thickness grafts consist of both the epidermis and the underlying dermis. The quality of skin following a full-thickness graft will be more natural than

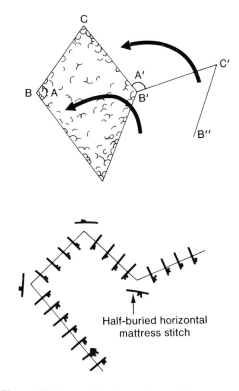

Figure 7-9 Transposition flap to close a diamond-shaped defect. Angle A′ = Angle A. B′ C′ = BC. B′ C′ = BD. *Source:* Reprinted from *Procedures and Techniques in Emergency Medicine* (p 300) by RR Simon and BE Brenner with permission of the Williams & Wilkins Company, Baltimore, © 1982.

that with a split-thickness graft. Full-thickness grafts are especially useful for repairing small defects in important parts of the body, such as avulsion injury to the tip of the nose. Generally speaking the donor site for a full-thickness graft must be undermined and closed primarily, or a deep scar will be left. Split-thickness grafts are useful for repairing large defects. The donor site regenerates a new epidermis from the remaining epidermal cells in the skin appendages.

Grafts, especially large grafts, are usually best referred to a surgeon.

Technique

The tissue is harvested from the donor site using a dermatome. The dermatome must be adjusted to yield the desired graft thickness. Graft donor sites should be in inconspicuous areas such as in the "panty area" of the buttocks. The medial aspect of the upper arm and the postauricular areas are useful donor sites for small full thickness grafts. One must be careful to match the characteristics of the donor and recipient sites as closely as possible in thickness, color, and texture. For example, never use a full-thickness graft from a hairy region to close a defect in a nonhairy region.

For large defects a split-thickness graft can be expanded to a larger size using a specialized mechanical device. With full-thickness grafts, all of the subcutaneous fat must be debrided from the bottom of the graft.

The skin graft should be placed so that it completely fills the defect. A graft that is too short results in a hematoma and pooling of fluid beneath the graft. Skin grafts rely on nutrients from the underlying tissue in order to survive. Thus a hematoma will cause the graft to necrose.

When suturing a graft in place, the suture material should pass through the graft first and then through the adjacent skin. Leave all of the suture ends quite long, and then use them to secure a stent (made by wrapping Xeroform gauze around fluffs of cotton) over the graft site, as shown in Figure 7-10. The stent reduces the risk of blood or serous fluid collecting beneath the graft. A firm pressure dressing can be used in lieu of or in addition to the buttress.

Whenever possible, elevation and immobilization are achieved during the first 7 to

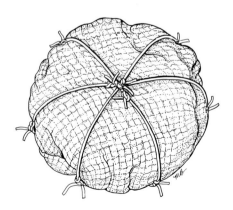

Figure 7-10 Skin graft dressing. A buttress consisting of Xeroform wrapped around cotton is secured using the free ends of the sutures used to stitch the graft to the skin.

10 days postoperatively. Dressing changes should *not* be performed for 4 or 5 days.

MARKEDLY IRREGULAR WOUND

General

Irregular wounds occur secondary to a number of mechanisms, including compression injuries such as the forehead striking the windshield, or when the cheek is struck by a fist or hard object. Irregular wounds are common in emergency departments, and therefore the emergency physician should become adept at their repair.

Repair Techniques

Elliptical Excision

Frequently the general shape of an irregular laceration is elliptical. In such cases, the irregularities can be excised with a simple arc on both sides of the wound and the resultant ellipse can be repaired in the standard manner.

W-Plasty

If marked irregularities are present, elliptical excision produces too wide a gap to close. Excellent results can be obtained by making several angled excisions and fitting together the two sides of the laceration somewhat like pieces in a puzzle (Fig. 7-11). The use of multiple linear débridement lines is termed a *W-plasty*.

Stellate Lacerations

Compression-type injuries, such as those resulting from striking the forehead against the ground, frequently lead to stellate lacerations with multiple converging flaps. With conventional suture techniques, the tips of the flaps frequently invert into the center of the wound. To avoid this problem, first use a half-buried horizontal mattress stitch to bring together all of the tips, and then repair the remainder of the laceration in the usual fashion (Fig. 7-12).

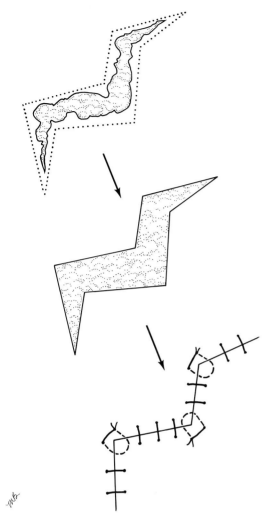

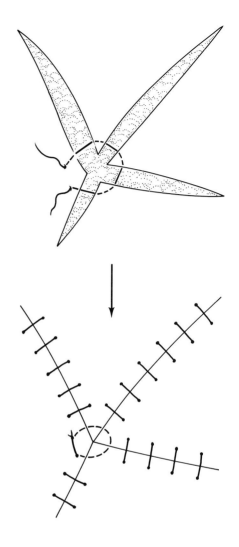

Figure 7-11 Repair of an irregular wound. Note that the corners are repaired using the half-buried horizontal mattress suture.

Figure 7-12 Repair of a stellate laceration using a half-buried horizontal mattress stitch.

For small stellate lesions, the best treatment is excision in order to yield an ellipse.

DOG-EAR DEFORMITIES

General

A *dog-ear deformity* is a pucker of tissue at one end of a sutured laceration that occurs because one edge exceeds the other in length. This disparity in lengths most often results from the extrinsic tension being greater on one side of the wound than the other, as well as with linear lacerations over a contoured area of the body such as the cheek.

As described in Chapter 5, the best way to avoid the dog ear deformity is to make minute adjustments during the repair, gathering slightly more tissue on the longer than the shorter side with each suture. Alternatively, one can close the wound by multiple bisecting stitches, also described in Chapter 5.

However, at times dog ears are unavoidable, especially in complex lacerations requiring rotation flaps.

Repair Techniques

Extend the Laceration

Direct extension of the laceration allows for the repair of the dog-ear deformity without any special maneuvers. After the direct extension, the sutures are placed taking care to gather slightly more tissue from the longer side, as shown in Figure 7-13.

Excision

A second, slightly more complicated means of repair involves slicing off a small triangle of tissue, as illustrated in Figure 7-14. This method is useful when the buckle is too great to be repaired by simple extension alone.

PARALLEL LACERATIONS

General

Parallel lacerations most commonly occur on the wrists, usually following a suicide attempt. These lacerations result in narrow strips of skin which must then be repaired.

Repair Techniques

Alternating Suture Placement

Staggered sutures through the central strip of skin alternately close the proximal and distal

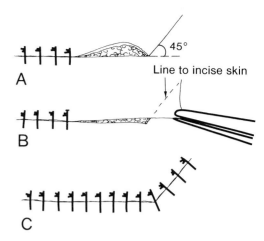

Figure 7-14 Dog-ear repair. With this technique, a small wedge is excised from one end of the wound. *Source*: Reprinted from *Procedures and Techniques in Emergency Medicine* (p 299) by RR Simon and P.E Brenner with permission of the Williams & Wilkins Company, Baltimore, © 1982.

lacerations, as shown in Figure 7-15. Note that the sutures are placed close to the wound edge, which helps to decrease the gaping that tends to occur when repairing parallel lacerations.

Modified Horizontal Mattress Suture

A horizontal mattress suture, which passes through the central skin strip in the subcuticular plane, is illustrated in Figure 7-16.

Skin Tape

Frequently skin tape alone can successfully close parallel lacerations (Fig. 7-17). Care should be taken not to let the tincture of benzoin come into contact with the subcutaneous tissue when painting the skin. The main problem encountered with this technique is that the skin of the volar wrist often inverts when closed with skin tape.

COMBINED LACERATION AND ABRASION

General

A combined abrasion and laceration occurs most frequently following a motorcycle or bicy-

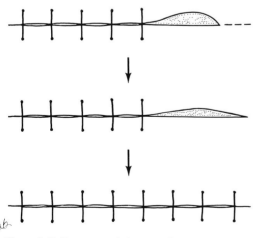

Figure 7-13 Dog-ear repair by extending the laceration. This method is especially useful for small tissue buckles.

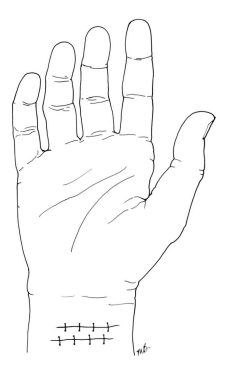

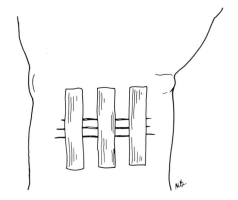

Figure 7-17 Skin tape closure of parallel lacerations.

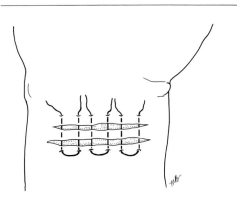

Figure 7-15 Parallel lacerations, staggered suture technique. The sutures in the central skin island alternate between the proximal and distal lacerations.

Figure 7-16 Repair of parallel lacerations using a modified horizontal mattress stitch. The hatched lines lie in the subcuticular plane.

cle accident. Broad areas of tissue can become abraded, and some tissue within the abrasion can rip, leading to a laceration as well. Using standard repair technique for the laceration is not possible, because the nonabsorbable skin sutures often become imbedded in the abrasion eschar as healing proceeds, especially if the patient is not

diligent about keeping the occlusive bandages in place.

Repair Technique

The wound should be cleaned, prepared, and anesthetized in the usual fashion. Then, instead of the usual skin closure, we recommend interrupted buried sutures of either Vycril or Dexon. The buried knot technique should be employed (see Chapter 5). Keep the top portion of the suture loop superficial, preferably in the subcuticular region, to insure alignment of the skin edges (Fig. 7-18). A standard subcuticular repair using absorbable sutures can also be employed. After the laceration has been closed, the wound should be dressed with an antibiotic ointment and covered with an occlusive bandage.

BEVELED EDGE LACERATIONS

General

Unlike the neat, 90 degree wound edges shown in Chapter 5 of this book, many of the lacerations the emergency physician encounters are cut on a tangent, yielding beveled edges. If such beveled wounds are sutured with a standard skin suture loop, an unsightly tissue ledge frequently results. Therefore, special techniques need to be applied to repair lacerations with beveled edges (see also Flap Lacerations, below).

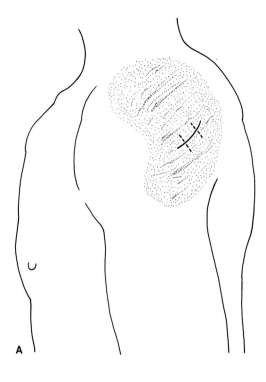

Taking a normal to somewhat generous bite from the broad edge, followed by a very small bite (2 mm from the edge) from the thin edge usually yields an excellent, level wound repair, as shown in Figure 7-19.

Debride the Edges

A second, more time-honored (but also time-consuming) method consists of debriding the edges to eliminate the beveled angles, as illustrated in Figure 7-20. The débridement technique is especially well suited to compression lacerations in which the tissue of the thin edge is macerated and would be prone to necrosis or infection.

Skin Tape

Shallow, beveled lacerations, especially when due to a shear injury, can be simply and acceptably repaired with skin tape.

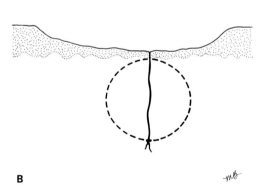

Figure 7-18 Repair of a laceration in abraded skin. Use an absorbable material such as Vycril. See text for discussion.

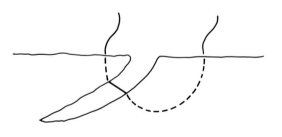

Repair Techniques

Small Bite from Thin Edge

One would think that taking a large bite from the thin edge and a tiny bite from the broad edge would help level out the repair. As it turns out, however, exactly the opposite strategy works.

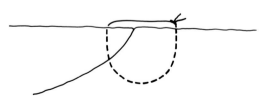

Figure 7-19 Repair of a beveled laceration. Taking a large bite from the large side and a small bite from the small side yields a level repair. Taking equal bites from the large side and the small side often results in a ledge.

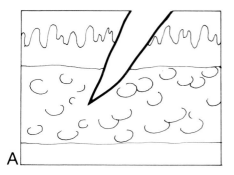

A

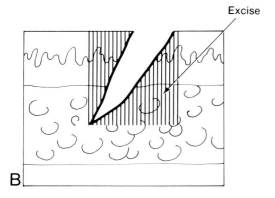

Excise

B

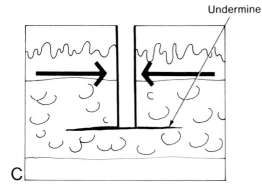

Undermine

C

Figure 7-20 Débridement of beveled edges. *Source:* Reprinted from *Procedures and Techniques in Emergency Medicine* (p 303) by RR Simon and BE Brenner with permission of the Williams & Wilkins Company, Baltimore, © 1982.

FLAP LACERATIONS

General

Many lacerations, particularly on the extremities, have a flap configuration. If the base of

the flap is proximal, it is termed a *proximal flap*. If the base of the flap is distal, it is termed a *distal flap*. Because proximal flaps possess a superior blood supply to distal ones, proximal flaps are less likely to necrose. Similarly, flaps in well-perfused regions, such as the face and scalp, heal better than those in poorly perfused regions, such as the lower extremities.

Flap Survival

The acceptable length/width ratios of flaps vary with the region of the body involved. For example, a distal flap that is two and a half times as long as it is wide may survive on the face but necrose on the foot (Table 7-1).

As a general rule, proximal flaps of the face and scalp with a length/width ratio of 3:1 survive. Proximal flaps of the trunk with a length/width ratio 1.5 to 2:1 survive. Proximal flaps of the distal extremities with a length/width ratio of 1 to 2:1 usually survive.

The survival rate is worse for transverse and distal flaps. The survival is also worse in areas of motion (such as extensor surface of joints) and in patients with poor perfusion (e.g., those with atherosclerosis or diabetes).

Flap Repair

Viable Flaps

Flaps that have adequate perfusion (see Flap Survival, above) should be tacked down with as

Table 7-1 Length/Width Ratios for Proximal Flaps

Location	Length/Width Ratio
Face and neck	3:1
Arm/forearm	1.5–2:1
Hand	2:1
Torso	2:1
Thigh/leg	1.5:1
Foot	1–1.5:1

few sutures as possible, keeping the sutures close to the edges to preserve perfusion. Be certain not to cinch the sutures down using too much tension, or perfusion to the flap will be compromised. The half-buried horizontal mattress suture is ideal for flap repairs, because the suture lies above the skin blood vessels (Fig. 7-21).

Flaps of Questionable Viability

When flaps are too long to have adequate perfusion of the tip, the flap should be trimmed to a smaller length before suturing (Fig. 7-22). Undermining will help to decrease the size of the

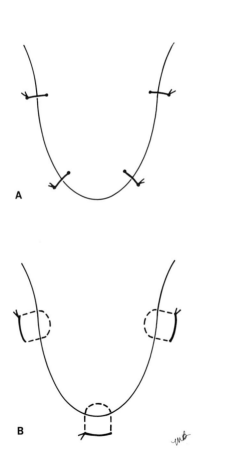

Figure 7-21 Flap lacerations. Flaps can be sutured down either using simple sutures (**A**) or half-buried horizontal mattress sutures (**B**).

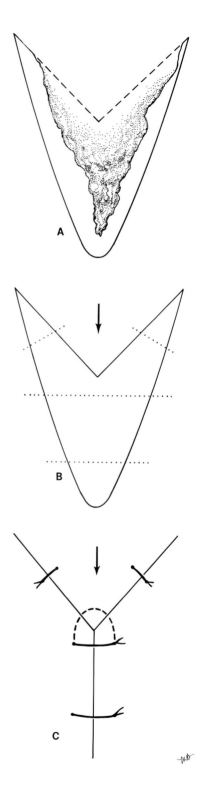

Figure 7-22 Flaps that are too long for survival should be trimmed and sutured. See text for discussion.

defect. Note that the central half-buried horizontal mattress stitch both positions the flap in place and decreases the size of the defect.

Small flaps can be entirely excised, leaving an elliptical defect that is closed in the usual manner.

An alternate method of repairing large nonviable flaps is to scrape the subcutaneous fat from beneath the flap and then tack down the flap (Fig. 7-23). Without the underlying fat, healing takes place in the same manner as for full-thickness skin grafts. As with full-thickness grafts, the wound should be covered with a stent.

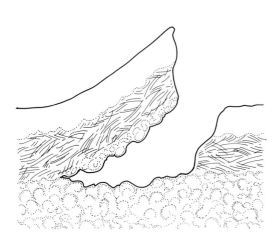

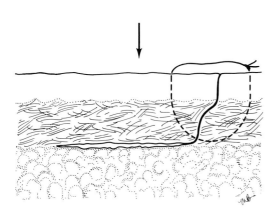

Figure 7-23 Repair of skin flaps that have inadequate blood supply for primary repair. The subcutaneous fat is scraped off and the flap is tacked down and allowed to heal in the same manner as a full-thickness skin graft.

Thin (Partial-Thickness) Flaps

Sometimes lacerations caused by knife wounds or glass cuts lead to thin flaps of skin consisting only of the epidermis and the superficial dermis. No subcutaneous fat can be seen.

If these thin flaps are sutured into place, survival of the flap usually occurs. However, the healed flap may become heaped up and edematous, especially on the extremities. Thus these small lesions are best treated by complete excision, covering the exposed defect with an occlusive dressing the same as for other split-thickness abrasions.

CONTAMINATED WOUNDS— DELAYED PRIMARY CLOSURE

General

The advantages of secondary closure (i.e., contaminated wounds that are left open are less prone to infection than those closed by primary intent) and primary closure can be joined by doing a *delayed primary closure*.

Technique

The wound is first irrigated and debrided, covered with a layer of Xeroform gauze and then the cavity filled with a bulky absorbent dressing. The wound should not be disturbed for 4 to 5 days. On the return visit, the wound is irrigated with normal saline and closed with single-layer of nylon or polypropylene sutures.

SCAR REVISION—THE Z-PLASTY

General

With healing, the resultant scar can lead to problems. For example, a scar that crosses perpendicular to a flexion crease of a joint can limit the range of motion of the joint. Scars that cross natural skin creases at the junctions of convexities and concavities (such as the nasolabial fold) can become thickened and unsightly. In such cases, the orientation of the scar can be revised using a Z-plasty.

Although some physicians favor use of the Z-plasty during the primary repair of lacerations that cross a flexor crease, in the authors' experience contractures develop in the minority as opposed to the majority of patients. The Z-plasty can thus be reserved for those who subsequently develop problems.

Technique

Two skin flaps are formed by incising the skin at 60 degree angles to the original laceration (or scar) as shown in Figure 7-24. These flaps are undermined and the position of each flap is transposed, so that the bottom flap moves to the top and vice versa. The result is a dramatic change in the orientation of the original scar line.

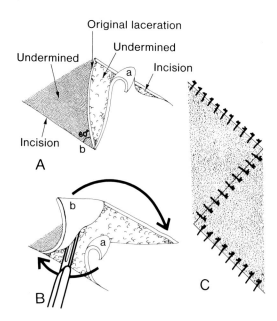

Figure 7-24 The Z-Plasty. See text for discussion. *Source:* Reprinted from *Procedures and Techniques in Emergency Medicine* (p 299) by RR Simon and BE Brenner with permission of the Williams & Wilkins Company, Baltimore, © 1982.

Chapter 8

Regional Care

This chapter presents the evaluation and treatment of wounds according to the region of the body that is injured. Table 8-1 lists suture materials for various regions. See Table 11-2 for time for suture removal.

THE SCALP

Anatomy

The scalp is well nourished by blood vessels that enter from the base of the scalp. The

supraorbital and supratrochlear arteries enter the scalp anteriorly; the superficial temporal and posterior auricular arteries enter the scalp laterally; and the occipital artery enters the scalp posteriorly. These vessels are relatively large and form an intercommunicating network which covers the entire scalp. It is because of this interconnecting network of arteries that hemorrhage from a laceration over the anterior portion of the scalp cannot be stopped by simply applying pressure over the supraorbital artery.

Arterial and venous plexi lie in the dermis of the scalp. The dermis of the scalp is one of the thickest in the body and is relatively inelastic. Thus, there is limited capability for elastic contraction of the skin of the scalp or for retraction of the arterioles in the dermis of the scalp. This relative inelasticity accounts for the marked tendency of scalp lacerations to bleed, even to the point of fatal exsanguination.

Evaluation

Prior to any evaluation of a scalp laceration, one must ascertain if there is ongoing bleeding. Controlling such bleeding can be difficult, particularly when one is dealing with macerated skin edges or an underlying hematoma. Many techniques are available for hemorrhage control. The first measure should be to place direct pres-

Table 8-1 Choice of Suture Materials

Site	Suture Material
Scalp	4-0 or 5-0 prolene or nylon, thin scalp 3-0 or 4-0 prolene or nylon, thick scalp
Face	
Skin closure	6-0 prolene or nylon
Deep layer	5-0 Vycril or Dexon
Mouth and tongue	5-0 Vycril or Dexon, or 4-0 or 5-0 plain or chromic gut
Neck	5-0 or 6-0 prolene or nylon
Trunk	4-0 or 5-0 prolene or nylon
Arm and leg	4-0 or 5-0 prolene or nylon
Palms and soles	4-0 or 5-0 prolene or nylon
Hand	5-0 or 6-0 prolene or nylon

sure with 4 inch × 4 inch gauze pads held in place for 10 to 15 minutes. The pads can be held down with an Ace bandage applied circumferentially around the scalp, or with direct pressure with a hand. If blood continues to soak through the gauze of the pressure dressing, the pack should be removed and the edges of the wound should be infiltrated with 1 percent lidocaine with epinephrine. In the special circumstance of a stellate laceration with macerated edges and an underlying hematoma, the infiltration of the Xylocaine with epinephrine should be deposited circumferentially about the entire wound. If arterioles at the wound edge continue to bleed, these can be clamped with a hemostat and ligated with Dexon or Vycril. If bleeding persists, 4 inch × 4 inch gauze pads soaked with 1:10,000 epinephrine can be applied to the wound and held in place with an Ace bandage.

The above techniques will control significant bleeding from most scalp lacerations. In instances where the hemorrhage persists despite these measures, a tourniquet should be placed around the entire scalp using either a large elastic drain held in place with a hemostat, or a strong, constricting rubber band. Remember that pressure over a single artery in the proximity of the wound is not sufficient, owing to the extensive arterial anastomoses.

After hemostasis is achieved, a thorough neurologic evaluation of the patient should be performed prior to any suture repair of a laceration. There are anecdotal reports of patients actually lapsing into comas and dying during repair of large scalp lacerations. The neurologic evaluation, and proper precautions for dealing with possible cervical spine injuries, are well described in general emergency medicine texts.[154]

In the evaluation of a scalp laceration, be certain to place a gloved finger into the wound in order to check for a palpable linear or depressed skull fracture. If a stellate laceration is present, the incidence of a fracture is much higher. If one does find an edge of a linear fracture, or a palpable depression, appropriate radiographs should be obtained. If a fracture is detected, do not palpate excessively within the wound as this can induce significant hemorrhage or cause dislodgment of a fracture fragment. If a fracture is documented, the patient should have the lacera-

tion treated as any open fracture by débridement and repair in the operating room.

Treatment

Basic Technique

Most scalp lacerations can be adequately repaired with a single-layer closure. Because the various layers of the scalp are adherent to one another, closing the uppermost layers will, at the same time, approximate the lower layers. Using a large needle allows for more of the layers to be encompassed in each suture loop. The loops should be cinched under slightly more tension than in other regions of the body because of the tendency of scalp lacerations to continue to bleed even after the sutures have been placed. When possible, a pressure dressing should be placed over the repaired area to decrease the risks of formation of a deep hematoma.

For extensive lacerations, the galea should be closed separately with interrupted absorbable sutures. Especially with large flap lacerations, if the galea is not closed separately retractions of the skin edges can occur during healing, resulting in a wider and thicker scar. This is especially a problem in men, who may develop balding. The top layer can then be closed using either a locked running suture, simple interrupted sutures, or vertical mattress sutures as indicated. The authors do not advocate using the horizontal mattress suture for scalp lacerations, as it does not offer as good approximation of the wound edges. This suture is reserved for patients in whom the edges are so macerated that they will not hold a conventional stitch (see Repair of an Irregular Scalp Laceration with Macerated Edges, below). The use of a pressure bandage is especially important in large lacerations, to prevent hematoma formation.

Closing a Defect

In the scalp, undermining should be performed below hair follicles in order to prevent bald spots from occurring due to destruction of follicles. The loose areolar tissue which is above the galea is the best natural plane.

In addition to, or instead of undermining, tension can be relieved when there is tissue loss in the scalp by "scoring" the galea, as illustrated in Figure 8-1. *Scoring* is a process in which linear slits are cut into the galea parallel to the laceration. This permits some opening to occur in the galea when one is approximating the wound edges, allowing for more relaxation of the skin above the area that has been scored.

Owing to the rich vascular supply of the scalp, the wound edges can be pulled together under more tension than would be tolerated in other parts of the body. Thus defects can be closed by approximating the edges with strong, broad sutures of 3-0 polypropylene or 3-0 nylon.

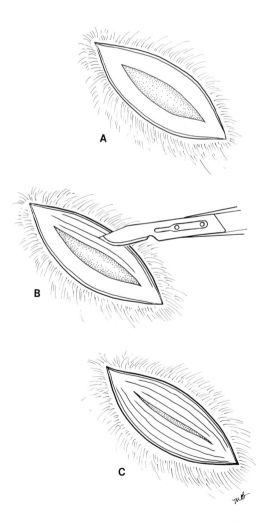

Figure 8-1 Scoring the galea. The scalpel makes linear, partial-thickness cuts in the galea (**B**). The result is a smaller gape in the wound (**C**).

Repair of a Laceration with an Underlying Hematoma

If the hematoma is deep to the laceration (e.g., subgaleal) and there is definitely no connection between the hematoma and the laceration (i.e., no possibility that the hematoma has been contaminated), the laceration can be repaired in the usual manner but without the use of deep sutures. A pressure dressing should be applied and the patient cautioned to sleep with the head elevated. The patient should be advised that a small nodule may form as residual fibrous tissue is deposited after the hematoma resolves.

If the laceration communicates with the hematoma space, the hematoma is contaminated and must be completely evacuated prior to wound closure. If this evacuation is not done, the hematoma is prone to becoming infected. After wound closure, a pressure dressing must be applied or the hematoma will reaccumulate. Some authorities advocate placing a drain in large spaces left following evacuation of hematomas but we have not found this necessary (see Chapter 5, Section Surgical Drains).

Repair of an Irregular Scalp Laceration with Macerated Edges

When wound edges are badly macerated, they should be trimmed minimally. Excessive trimming of a scalp laceration can make subsequent closure impossible. The skin should then be approximated using large bites with a horizontal mattress suture which allows for approximation of the edges without having to pass a suture into the macerated and "soupy" tissue (Fig. 8-2). Due to the rich vasculature of the scalp, the infection rate of macerated lacerations is surprisingly low.

Scalp Avulsion

Severe head injuries can lead to the avulsion of all or part of the scalp. In some cases microsurgical reanastomosis of the blood vessels to the avulsed tissue can make reimplantation possible.[175] Therefore the avulsed tissue should be cleansed, wrapped in saline-soaked gauze, placed in a plastic bag, and cooled pending consultation with an appropriate specialist.

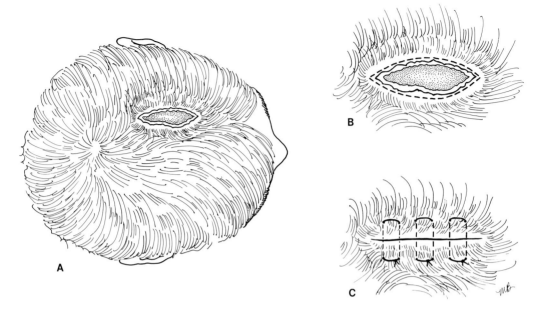

Figure 8-2 Repair of macerated scalp laceration with macerated edges (**A**). **B.** The edges are trimmed minimally. **C.** The wound is then closed using a horizontal mattress stitch. The horizontal mattress stitch is reserved for lacerations with macerated edges.

THE FACE

General

Lacerations and Abrasions

All the techniques of plastic tissue repair come into play when repairing facial lacerations. Abrasions should be cleansed of any foreign material to avoid permanent tattooing. Irregular edges of lacerations should be trimmed prior to suturing.

The tissue should be handled with the utmost care and gentleness to keep scarring to a minimum. Skin hooks are frequently useful in this regard.

Lacerations that gape or that enter deeply into the dermis should be repaired with a layered closure technique. If the deep tissue is not repaired, the scar will have the potential for widening with time, causing an unacceptable cosmetic result. The deep layer(s) can be repaired with 4-0 or 5-0 Dexon or Vycril, using the buried knot technique (see Chapter 5).

The skin should be closed using a fine suture material such as 6-0 polypropylene or nylon. In some cases the synthetic materials tend to distort the skin, for example, on the upper eyelid. In such cases 6-0 silk can be used instead, although it is more reactive than synthetic suture materials. Alternatively, one can use polypropylene or nylon, using an open-loop knot (see Chapter 6). The sutures should be placed 1 to 2 mm from the wound edge, and 2 to 3 mm apart.

Both lacerations and abrasions should be covered with either an occlusive dressing (such as polyurethane film) or an antimicrobial ointment, both of which inhibit crusting. If an ointment is used, caution the patient to reapply it every 4 to 6 hours until suture removal for lacerations, or until the wound has healed for abrasions. If a crust forms over the wound, not only is suture removal more tedious and difficult, but epithelialization is retarded and the degree of scarring may actually be increased (see Chapter 11).

Skin sutures should be removed early: in 3 to 4 days in children, and 4 to 5 days in adults. Following suture removal skin tape should be used for approximately 10 to 14 days to provide additional support for the healing wound. Since the epidermis is healed, non-sterile tape will suffice.

Tissue Loss in Facial Lacerations

Lost tissue can be recovered, and if not severely traumatized, it should be defatted and used as a full-thickness graft. This permits the best possible results when too much tissue is lost for primary closure to be possible. If the defects are large, a free skin graft or a flap will be necessary, which are best done by a plastic surgeon. Some avulsions are best treated by allowing the defect to heal in by secondary intent, letting normal wound contraction occur, and then performing elective scar revision.

As with the scalp, microvascular surgery can make possible the reimplantation of parts of the face that have been avulsed, such as the ear. Therefore, avulsed tissue should be cleansed, wrapped in saline-soaked gauze, placed in a plastic bag, and kept cool.

The Forehead

Anatomy

The forehead is traversed by the supraorbital and supratrochlear arteries and nerves. Large hematomas can thus form following a forehead contusion. Lacerations of the forehead can be associated with significant bleeding; however, such bleeding is easier to control than with scalp lacerations because of the ability of the dermis and the dermal arterioles to contract.

In repairing lacerations of the forehead, one must keep in mind that the relaxed skin tension lines in this region are oriented horizontally.

Evaluation

As with any head injury, the patient should be evaluated for possible associated neurologic or cervical spine injuries. Patients who sustain forehead lacerations by striking an automobile windshield should be checked for retained particles of glass prior to closing the lacerations. Surprisingly large glass fragments can underlie even small skin punctures owing to the elasticity of the tissues.

Treatment

Lacerations, General Considerations. Look at the direction of the laceration in relation to the skin tension lines. Lacerations running perpendicular to the tension lines can be closed primarily, but the patient should be advised that a poor scar may result if contraction occurs. The orientation of a curvilinear or U-shaped laceration can at times be changed with minimal effort to produce a much better cosmetic result. This is discussed in U-shaped flaps, below.

U-Shaped Flaps. U-shaped flaps can occur when patients strike their forehead against an automobile windshield. The shattering of glass causes fragments to be imbedded under a flap of tissue. Hence, such lesions should be probed and these glass fragments should be removed.

Small (4 to 5 mm) flaps that are well perfused and not shaved at a tangent can be simply tacked down with a single interrupted skin suture as shown in Figure 8-3. Flaps in which the skin edges naturally touch even before any repair is undertaken do especially well with the single-stitch technique. The half-buried horizontal mattress stitch is also useful in U-flap repair.

U-shaped flaps that tend to retract, leaving a defect, and U-flaps that appear ischemic at the distal segment often heal in a bunched-up, raised fashion called a "biscuit deformity." In such

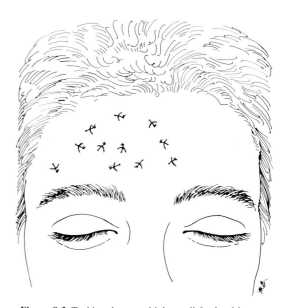

Figure 8-3 Tacking down multiple small forehead lacerations resulting from striking an automobile windshield. Prior to suturing, each laceration should be probed for retained glass fragments.

cases, excision of the entire flap leaving an ellipse that runs parallel to the skin tension lines can be performed, as shown in Figure 8-4.

Large Flaps and Lacerations. Large forehead flaps are irrigated and prepped in the usual fashion. The wound edges are trimmed in the usual manner, using either a sharp iris scissors or scalpel. The wound is undermined in the subcutaneous plane. Next, the frontalis muscle fascia and the subcutaneous tissue should be repaired in separate layers, using absorbable sutures with the buried knot technique (see Chapter 5). The skin is then carefully closed using polypropylene or nylon. The sutures should be removed in 4 days, and skin tape applied for an additional 10 to 14 days.

In general, large excisions of tissue to realign a laceration to lie parallel to the skin tension lines should not be done as part of the emergency department repair procedure. Such excisions can lead to a permanent upward tenting of the ipsilateral eyebrow, as shown in Figure 8-5.[96] The scar can then be electively revised by a plastic surgeon after the wound has healed and remodeled, in 6 to 8 months.

Stellate Lacerations. Stellate lacerations can be repaired using the half-buried horizontal mattress stitch described in Chapter 6. Stellate lacerations that are badly macerated result in a poor scar which may require later revision. If the stellate laceration is small, and can be excised within the lines of skin tension, this is preferred.

Tissue Defects. A small tissue defect of less than 2 to 3 cm can often be closed by undermining and advancing the adjacent tissues. Larger defects require advanced techniques such as grafting or rotation flaps and generally should be referred to a plastic surgeon (see Chapter 7).

Forehead Hematomas. Large forehead hematomas should be drained and the area covered with a pressure dressing. If the hematoma is not drained, an unsightly nodule of fibrous tissue can result.

Complex Forehead Abrasions. Deep abrasions with ground-in road dirt are a frequent problem for the emergency specialist. In addition to being abraded, the skin frequently contains numerous small, parallel lacerations.

Road dirt and particulate matter left embedded in the wound result in permanent pigmentation as the particles are phagocytosed by tissue macrophages. This process begins to occur within 72 hours after the injury. Thus, particulate matter must be removed as soon after the injury as possible.

Anesthesia for cleansing a complex forehead abrasion is best performed using supraorbital nerve blocks (see Chapter 3). When this is not possible, topical anesthesia can be obtained by holding gauze soaked with 4 percent lidocaine over the region for 15 to 20 minutes.

The area is then irrigated under pressure using a 35-cc syringe and an 18-gauge angiocath. Remaining imbedded material can be removed by rubbing the region with a saline-soaked gauze or by using the tip of a no. 11 scalpel blade to tease out debris.

A dry dressing permits desiccation of the superficial dermis. In cases where there is residual pigment retained in this superficial der-

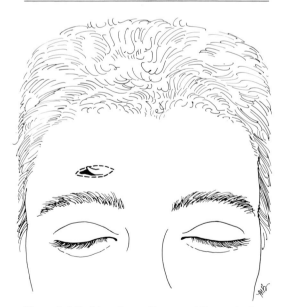

Figure 8-4 Excision of a small, retracted flap on the forehead. The excision is made along the natural skin tension lines. See text for discussion.

Figure 8-5 Débridement of forehead lacerations. **A.** A large, angulated forehead laceration. **B1.** Débridement following the major lines of the laceration. **B2.** The entire laceration is excised, leaving a gaping ellipse. **C1.** With conservative débridement a small scar is left, but the orientation of the eyebrows is normal. **C2.** Following the wide, elliptical excision, the scar line itself is less noticeable but the ipsilateral brow is tented up in a disfiguring manner. ⟶

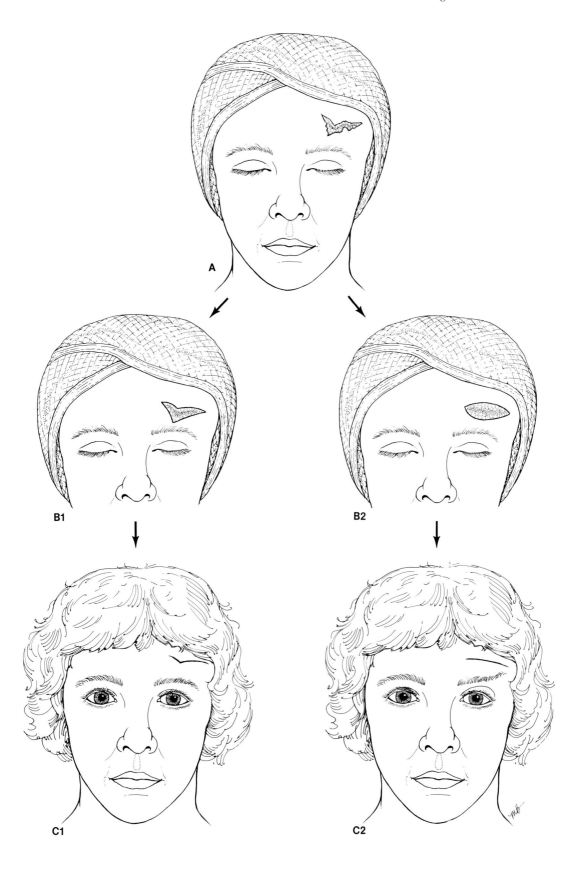

A

B1   B2

C1   C2

mis despite vigorous efforts outlined above, allowing the wound to dry causes some of the discolored dermis to be incorporated into the eschar, which then peels away as epithelialization ensues. In cases where the abrasion can be debrided of all imbedded material, an occlusive dressing (such as polyurethane film) or ointment should be used to cover the wound, since occlusive dressings speed the healing of abrasions (see Chapter 11).

When lacerations are present within the abrasion, these can be repaired using shallow, subcutaneous buried-knot sutures of 5-0 Dexon or Vycril (see Chapter 7). The edges of badly macerated lacerations should be excised. At times, multiple parallel lacerations in close proximity to one another can be excised to yield a single laceration.

The Periorbital Region

Anatomy

The relaxed skin tension lines are oriented circumferentially around the eye, conforming to the orbicularis oculi muscle. The eyelids contain a tarsal plate, which is a fibrocartilaginous structure providing support to the upper lids. The medial canthus is generally speaking a "no-man's land" for the emergency physician, because of the presence of the lacrimal apparatus in this region. Thus a laceration involving the medial canthus should generally be repaired by a plastic surgeon or ophthalmologist.

Evaluation

In evaluating lacerations of the periorbital skin and eyelids one must first evaluate the eye itself. Penetrating and blunt injuries to the eyelids and periorbital skin can be associated with major injuries to the globe and cornea with little clinical evidence at the onset. Therefore, always do a careful eye examination, including visual acuity, slit lamp, eversion of the upper lid to look for a foreign body, and examination of the cornea (with fluorescence if there is risk of a corneal abrasion), transillumination of the anterior chamber to check for hyphema, and a funduscopic retinal examination. The extraocular muscles should be evaluated. Loss of upgaze signals the presence of an orbital blowout fracture. If the visual fields are not intact, the patient should be referred for indirect ophthalmoscopy to check for a retinal detachment. Unlike spontaneous detachments, traumatic retinal detachments frequently remain asymptomatic for several hours or even days due to sparing of the macula.

Any lid laceration involving the medial canthus must be evaluated for a possible injury to the lacrimal apparatus. The integrity of the duct can be verified by instilling fluorescein into the eye and checking with a Wood's lamp for the presence of fluorescein in the nasal secretions. Because this examination cannot screen for partial lacrimal duct lacerations, deep lacerations in the medial canthal region should usually be referred to a plastic surgeon or ophthalmologist.

When a patient's history suggests that an eye laceration may have been caused by a metallic foreign body, then a radiograph of the globe should be done to ascertain whether there is a foreign body within the globe. CT scan and ultrasound can be used to detect non-metallic objects.

Lacerations of the upper lid should be carefully explored to determine whether the tarsal plate has been injured. In addition, the physician should gently explore lacerations of the periorbital skin to determine if there has been penetration into the orbit itself. If a circumferential hematoma completely covering the sclera is noted, rupture of the globe must be strongly suspected. However, similar hematomas occur in orbital fractures without rupture of the globe.

Axiom: A circumferential hematoma completely covering the sclera with no sclera visible is indicative of a rupture of the globe until proven otherwise. Rupture should also be suspected when there is enophthalmos or distortion of the globe.

When a globe rupture is diagnosed or suspected, the eye should be protected with a hard shield and the patient should be referred to a specialist. Never place a pressure patch over the eye if there is a question of a globe laceration.

When swelling and ecchymosis of the periorbital tissues prevent the patient from being able to open his or her eye, the lids should be opened with lid retractors and the eye examined for extraocular movements, possible hyphema, pupillary reaction, and if possible, acuity and funduscopic examination. If the initial examination is normal, the patient should still be instructed to return either to the emergency department or to go to an ophthalmologist in 3 to 4 days for a repeat examination when the swelling has subsided. Especially important at the follow-up examination is the visual field check.

Treatment

General. Wounds in the periorbital region pose special problems because of the need to avoid causing irritation to the eye during repair. Thus, wound preparation near the eye necessitates that no harsh prep solutions, such as isopropyl alcohol or surgical scrub detergents, be used to prepare the intact skin. It is safe to use saline to irrigate the wound, however. Be sure that a high-pressure irrigant stream is not allowed to strike the globe itself. A 1:10 dilution of povidone-iodine solution (*not* the irritating detergent scrub) may safely be used as a topical antiseptic for wounds in the vicinity of the eyes. In fact, some ophthalmologists recommend using this solution to irrigate the eye itself prior to ophthalmic surgery.[23]

When suturing tissue near the eye, be absolutely certain to keep the tip of the needle clear of the globe at all times.

Complex Eyebrow Lacerations. In repairing eyebrow lacerations, one must be careful to do minimal débridement. If débridement is necessary, for example, in a badly macerated laceration, excision should be carried out at an oblique angle so as not to cut across the hair follicles, which would result in bald spots (Fig. 8-6). The subcutaneous sutures should be carefully placed, so that once the deep layer is in the eyebrow naturally comes together without any skewing of its natural line. The skin should then be approximated with 6-0 nylon or polypropylene.

Lacerations of the Eyelids. The tissue of the eyelids is unique, being devoid of the usual layer of subcutaneous fat cells. The tissue of the upper lid is redundant, thus allowing for primary closure of small avulsions of tissue with good cosmetic results.

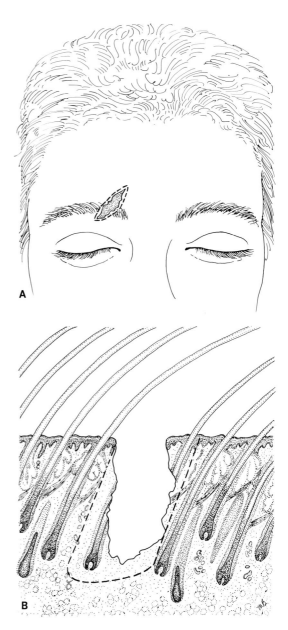

Figure 8-6 A and **B.** Débridement of a macerated eyebrow laceration. Débridement should be carried out at an oblique angle to avoid cutting across hair follicles and leaving a bald spot.

If fat is seen protruding through a laceration to the lid, this can often represent herniation from adipose tissue in the orbit itself, and the patient should be referred to an ophthalmologist.[45]

Simple lid lacerations are treated by direct approximation. The stitches should be placed just a few millimeters from the wound edge and should be only a few millimeters deep. Be especially careful not to penetrate the entire thickness of the lid, thereby risking penetration of the globe with the needle.

For lacerations that involve the lash-bearing lid margins, special care must be taken in the repair (Fig. 8-7). First, a suture is placed at the lid "gray line," between the lashes and the mucosa. Second, the tarsal plate is repaired with 5-0 Vycril or Dexon, using a buried knot deep suture. Third, the skin is closed using 6-0 nylon or polypropylene. If the laceration is extensive enough, another layer of fine Vycril or Dexon must be used to repair the palpebral conjunctiva.

Full-thickness lid lacerations that involve tissue loss (i.e., there is a notch of tissue missing from the lid margin) or that require more than minimal débridement are best referred to a plastic surgeon or ophthalmologist, unless the emergency physician has extensive experience in such repairs. Such lacerations frequently heal with permanent notching of the lid margin, even with the most careful repairs.

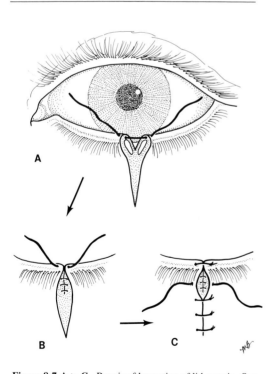

Figure 8-7 A to **C.** Repair of laceration of lid margin. See text for discussion.

The Cheek

Anatomy and Evaluation

The cheek has several important structures that affect the evaluation and repair of lacerations in this region. The facial nerve exits from beneath the parotid gland and its branches course just above the masseters and the muscles of facial expression. Hence, any laceration that penetrates to these muscles must be evaluated for injury to a branch of the facial nerve.

The physician must consider the muscles of facial expression when dealing with deep lacerations. The authors advise consulting a standard anatomy text when dealing with a facial laceration involving these muscles so as to ascertain which muscle is involved and to determine the orientation of the repair. The face should be carefully observed while the patient varies his or her facial expressions to ascertain whether asymmetry is present. Check for integrity of the muscles of facial expression *prior* to instilling local anesthetics, as anesthetics can cause temporary dysfunction of the 7th nerve.

Specialized septa attach to the dermis from the fascia of the muscles of expression, so undermining should be kept to a minimum to avoid damaging these important attachments.

Also of importance in the cheek is the parotid duct, which courses midway between the angle of the jaw and the zygomatic arch. An injury to this duct must be considered whenever one sees a laceration in this region. By means of a thorough exploration of the wound, possibly with an assistant retracting the tissue, the physician can usually ascertain if this injury has occurred. In addition, the physician can perform an intraoral examination to see if blood can be expressed from the orifice of the parotid duct (adjacent to the first molar) when the parotid gland is stroked. If blood comes from the orifice this indicates that the gland or duct has been lacerated.

The physician should pull the maxilla forward by exerting pressure with the thumb placed on the hard palate just behind the front incisors. Motion of the maxilla when this maneuver is performed indicates a LeFort facial fracture.

Depending on the mechanism of injury and the degree of swelling present, facial radiographs can be taken to check for fractures. Fractures that cause facial deformity or that interfere with the extraocular muscles should be referred to a specialist for definitive care. In most cases, the repair of facial fractures can be delayed for several days to allow for the swelling to subside.

Treatment

General. Always repair cheek lacerations with a layer-by-layer closure. This is vitally important due to the septal connections between the skin and the muscles of facial expression. Fine Vycril or Dexon can be employed for repair of deep layers.

Débridement. In the region of the lower eyelid, one must be careful to keep débridement to a minimum to avoid an ectropion (downward distortion) of the lid (Fig. 8-8).

As with all facial lacerations, the tissue should be handled with the utmost care and gentleness to keep scarring to a minimum. Skin hooks are frequently useful in this regard.

Lacerations That Cross Natural Concavities or Convexities. Certain lacerations cross natural concavities or convexities as shown in Figure 8-9. During the initial repair place the deep sutures in the usual manner. For the skin closure, however, it is essential that the accentuated lines be aligned exactly. To insure exact alignment the first suture should be placed at the accented skin tension line. For example, for the skin closure of a laceration that crosses the nasolabial fold, place the initial suture at the fold line. The remainder of the skin sutures are then placed in the usual manner.

If there is contraction of the scar as the wound heals, contortion of the accented skin lines occurs. Some practitioners recommend performing a Z-plasty at the primary repair, to reorient the scar to follow the accented skin lines (see Chapter 7, Section Z-Plasty). However, in the authors' experience, such contractures occur only in the minority of patients. Those in whom contraction occurs can be referred to a plastic surgeon for scar revision on an elective basis.

Through-and-Through Cheek Lacerations. The laceration should be closed in layers, beginning with the mucosa and ending with the skin. 5-0 Vycril or Dexon are useful sutures for the mucosa, because they are soft when moist

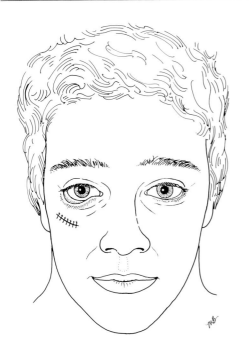

Figure 8-8 Overzealous débridement of upper cheek laceration leading to ectropion of the eyelid.

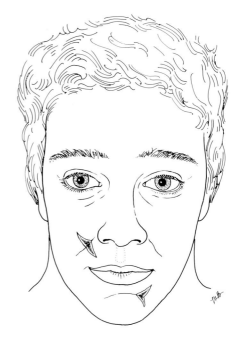

Figure 8-9 Lacerations crossing concavities or convexities.

(hence comfortable for the patient) and cause less of a reaction than chromic or plain gut. However, both Vycril and Dexon must be removed because they can take weeks to absorb on their own. The mucosal tissues should be approximated without undue tension. Enough sutures should be placed so that there are no gaps for saliva to seep through. The mucosa should be tested to be sure that a watertight seal has been obtained. This can be accomplished by irrigating a stream of saline against the mucosa and seeing if it leaks across.

After the mucosa is repaired, reirrigate the laceration with saline and prep the laceration itself, as well as the surrounding skin, with 1 percent povidone-iodine solution.

If the masseter muscle is lacerated, it should be repaired with 5-0 Dexon or Vycril placed through the muscle sheath. Next close the subcutaneous tissue, using either 5-0 Vycril or Dexon, with a buried knot suture. Finally, complete the closure with 6-0 nylon or polypropylene.

See Oral Cavity, below, regarding the use of prophylactic antibiotics.

The Lips

Anatomy

The lip is made up of two epithelial tissues which represent a transition between the oral mucosa and the skin. The point of this transition is called the *vermilion border*. The lip contains the orbicularis oris muscle, which must be repaired as a separate layer when lacerations involve this muscle.

Treatment

General. The main point to remember concerning the repair of lip lacerations is that the vermilion border must be lined up as exactly as possible. Malalignment by only 1 millimeter can be noticeable. A good way to avoid malalignment is to place the first skin suture at the vermilion border, aligning it exactly, and then proceed with the repair (Fig. 8-10). Figure 11-5 shows the finished repair (in Chapter 11, Aftercare).

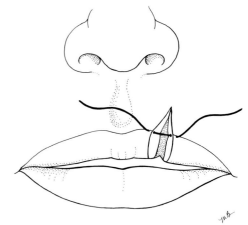

Figure 8-10 Placement of the initial stitch at the vermilion border during repair of lip laceration.

The tissue of the lips is somewhat spongy and often swells greatly when local anesthetics are instilled. Therefore, a regional block (infraorbital or mental nerves) is preferred over local infiltration for local anesthesia.

Through-and-Through Lip Lacerations. Through-and-through lip lacerations risk complication by saliva from the oral cavity entering and contaminating the wound. Although several techniques are available for repairing such lesions, the authors recommend the following method.

First, irrigate the wound with normal saline. The laceration should be closed in layers, beginning with the wet mucosa. 5-0 Vycril or Dexon are useful sutures for the mucosa because they are soft when moist (hence comfortable for the patient) and cause less of a reaction than chromic or plain gut. The mucosal tissues should be approximated without undue tension. Enough sutures should be placed so that there are no gaps for saliva to seep through.

After the wet mucosa is repaired, place a sterile gauze between the teeth and the lips, and reirrigate the laceration with saline, and then prepare the laceration itself as well as the surrounding skin with 1 percent povidone-iodine. Then drape the area, taking care not to obstruct breathing.

Next, place a single 6-0 polypropylene or nylon skin stitch through the vermilion border to insure its proper alignment (see above). This skin stitch should be left untied to facilitate placement of the deep sutures.

After the vermilion border suture has been placed, proceed with the deep sutures. If the orbicularis oris muscle is lacerated it should be repaired with 5-0 Dexon or Vycril. Next close the subcutaneous tissue, using 5-0 Vycril or Dexon, with a buried knot suture.

After the deep sutures are in place, tie the vermilion border suture and complete the closure of both the skin and the dry mucosa of the lip with 6-0 nylon or polypropylene. The skin is then dressed with an antibiotic ointment. The patient should return in 4 days for removal of the sutures.

See Oral Cavity, below, regarding the use of prophylactic antibiotics.

Lip Amputations. A small defect with tissue loss of less than 1½ cm can be closed primarily after débridement of the skin edges and careful approximation of the layers as described above. The lower lip especially is able to accommodate small avulsions with excellent cosmetic results.

We recommend that larger tissue avulsions be referred to a plastic surgeon for definitive care. Some plastic surgeons attempt reimplantation of avulsed segments, so these segments should be saved, as described above for scalp avulsions. Unfortunately, large avulsions, such as often occur following animal and human bites, often heal with poor cosmetic results even with the best of therapy.

The Oral Cavity

Anatomic Considerations

The oral cavity has three types of tissue, each of which must be considered separately when treating injuries: gingiva, buccal and palatal mucosa, and tongue.

Evaluation

Lacerations that involve the buccal mucosa must be evaluated for injury to the parotid duct when they occur in the vicinity of this duct. Lacerations to the floor of the mouth must be carefully evaluated for possible involvement of

the other salivary glands and of the ducts of these glands. When dealing with an injury to the gingiva, be certain that the tooth is not fractured below the gum line. If the tooth is tender to percussion or is loosened, obtain dental films to rule out possible fracture.

Axiom: A tooth that is tender to percussion, although appearing normal, should be thought of as having a fracture below the gum line until proven otherwise.

Treatment

Prophylactic Antibiotics. The use of prophylactic antibiotics for lacerations involving the oral cavity is frequently advised by both emergency physicians and oral surgeons. As with many issues of wound management, there have been no definitive studies to date to indicate whether or not such therapy is justified. However, studies do indicate that in the experimental animal antibiotics are efficacious only if given no later than 3 hours after the lacerations.[52]

The authors routinely use prophylactic antibiotics for intraoral lacerations, pending evidence to the contrary. The drug of choice is penicillin. Because the efficacy of prophylactic antibiotics is dependent on their being given as soon as possible after the wound is incurred, we recommend that the first dose be given when the patient is first seen, and not be delayed until after suturing, or worse yet until the patient leaves the hospital and fills the prescription.

For severe oral injuries, we administer the first dose as penicillin G, 1 million units IM or IV, followed by 500 mg penicillin V PO qid for 4 days. For routine cases, we give the first dose as oral penicillin 500 mg, followed by the same dose qid for 4 days.

Mucosal Lacerations. Mucosal lacerations less than 1 cm in length and not through-and-through usually do not open widely enough to require any repair. These lacerations seal within 12 hours and are well apposed, though not entirely healed, within 4 to 5 days.

The physician can close large or gaping lacerations with a single layer, using just enough stitches to bring the edges into apposition. Closure can be with either 4-0 plain gut, 5-0 silk, or 5-0 Vycril or Dexon. Silk sutures require a return visit for removal. In animal studies, Vycril and Dexon appear to be less pyogenic than silk or plain gut.[1,3,50,123,164,176] We recommend plain saline rinses of the mouth for aftercare, rather than more irritating solutions.

Tongue Lacerations. Tongue lacerations that are nongaping, and less than 1 cm in length, heal well without suturing, even in the case of through-and-through lesions. Large lacerations and gaping lacerations require suturing, as do U-shaped flaps, which can heal in an elevated fashion unless repaired. Just a few sutures to bring the tissue into apposition are required, using the same suture materials listed above for mucosal lacerations.

The physician may attempt to suture pediatric tongue lacerations in the emergency department, but in some patients this is impossible and repair under general anesthesia is necessary. Sedation is usually required to repair a laceration in a child. A bite block fashioned of 4 inch × 4 inch gauze pads wrapped around two tongue blades and fixed in place with adhesive tape can be wedged between the molars to keep the mouth open. In addition, a suture can be passed through the tip of the tongue using 2-0 silk in order to retract the tongue while doing the repair. This suture is removed when the repair is completed.

Gingival Lacerations. Lacerations involving the gingiva require special considerations. Small lacerations can be repaired in the normal fashion. Since plain gut can be irritating to the gingiva, the authors prefer to use Vycril, silk, or Dexon. As was true for mucosal lacerations, both Vycril and Dexon can take weeks to be absorbed and thus require removal. Anesthesia with viscous lidocaine is frequently sufficient.

The gingiva has no subcutaneous support, hence when a flap-type laceration occurs it ''flops'' open (Fig. 8-11A). This poses a difficult treatment problem. Repair by simple approximation does not suffice. Repair should be accomplished making a stitch that runs circumferentially around the tooth as illustrated in Figure 8-11B and C. Be certain that the circumferential suture loops are not so tight as to strangulate the tissues.

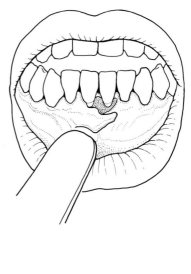

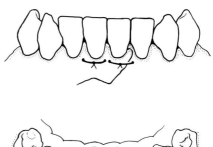

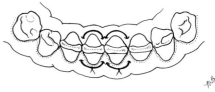

Figure 8-11 A. Gingival open flap laceration. **B.** Front view of repair. **C.** Cross-section of repair. See text for discussion.

Hard Palate Lacerations. Lacerations of the hard palate can be loosely approximated, using the same suture materials listed for mucosal lacerations, and heal well. These lacerations are frequently due to impalement against the end of a firm object. For small lacerations, in which the edges appose well naturally, no suturing is necessary.

In dealing with large lacerations in children, sedation is almost always necessary. Then, 4 inch × 4 inch gauze pads wrapped around a tongue blade lodged between the molars make an excellent bite block to keep the oral cavity open.

Soft Palate Lacerations. With impalement injuries to the soft palate, one must keep in mind that the impaling object may have passed posteriorly to strike and then lacerate the posterior pharyngeal wall (see Posterior Pharynx Lacerations, below). If a high posterior pharynx laceration is possible, then the patient should be referred to an ear, nose, and throat (ENT) physician for further evaluation.

Lacerations to the soft palate in which the base of the wound is completely intact (and hence there is no possibility that the posterior nasal pharynx was also impaled) can be treated in the same manner as the hard palate. Deep soft palate lacerations can extend to the deep tissue planes of the neck and even to the carotid artery, and therefore require referral to an ENT specialist.

Posterior Pharyngeal Lacerations. Lacerations involving the posterior pharynx most commonly result from impalement on a firm object. A common scenario is a child who runs with a toothbrush in his or her mouth and then falls, impaling the toothbrush against the back of the throat.

Patients with significant (i.e., cutting all the way through the mucosa) posterior pharyngeal lacerations require immediate ENT referral for admission and parenteral antibiotics. They should be kept NPO (in case operative repair is required) and the first doses of antibiotics (one of which should be high-dose penicillin G) should be given in the emergency department.

The seriousness of this seemingly innocent laceration stems from the fact that there is a fascial plane (the so-called "space of danger") underlying the posterior pharyngeal mucosa which is continuous with the fascial planes of the mediastinum. Thus an infection in the region of a posterior pharyngeal laceration can progress into fatal mediastinitis.

Axiom: *An infection of a posterior pharyngeal laceration can progress to mediastinitis.*

The Ear[45]

Anatomy

The cartilaginous portions of the ear are adherent to the skin. In these areas there is virtually no subcutaneous tissue. Hematomas in this area are associated with deposition of fibrous tissue, which with repeated episodes brings about the unsightly "cauliflower ear" deformity. The exact names of the various portions of the external ear become important when one is documenting the exact nature of an auricular laceration (Fig. 8-12).

Evaluation

Inspect and then palpate the auricle for hematomas. Check for blood behind the tympanic membrane. A hemotympanum signifies a basilar skull fracture, even if the plain skull films appear to be normal. Evaluate if there is any tissue loss in a badly macerated ear.

Treatment[115]

Ear Lacerations (Cartilage Spared). The ear should be cleaned and prepared in the usual fashion. Cotton-tipped applicators are useful to prepare hard-to-reach convolutions.

Débridement should be done only to remove skin that is clearly nonviable. The excellent blood supply of the face allows for survival of thin flaps of skin that in other parts of the body would necrose within hours.

The wound edges in ear lacerations have a tendency to invert; if this is allowed to happen, an unsightly, permanent ridge in the tissue forms. Therefore, when repairing a laceration over the cartilaginous portion of the ear, be certain to take small bites (i.e., 1 to 2 mm from the

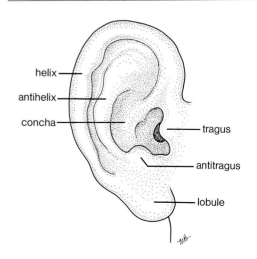

Figure 8-12 The anatomy of the external ear.

wound edge) in order to avoid inversion of the skin. In some cases, shallow vertical mattress sutures (keeping clear of the underlying cartilage) must be alternated with the simple ties to overcome the tendency of the skin edges to invert.

When repairing ear lacerations, the physician should make certain that no areas of cartilage are left uncovered by skin. Cartilage exposed to air can develop a chronic chondritis that is difficult to treat.

For small lacerations frequent application of an antibiotic ointment suffices for the wound dressing. Extensive lacerations require a compressive dressing (see Compressive Dressing, below). Sutures can be removed in 4 to 5 days for adults and 3 to 4 days for children. When possible, skin tapes should be placed following suture removal.

Wounds Involving the Cartilage. When cartilage is lacerated or abraded, it should be thoroughly cleansed by saline lavage, followed by direct preparation with dilute povidone-iodine solution. Débridement of cartilage should be extremely conservative, and only grossly necrotic tissue should be excised. The wound edge that results should be such that the skin overlies the cartilage by about 1 mm. If the skin extends slightly beyond the cartilage in the wound edge this facilitates eversion when the skin is closed. Therefore, if the cartilage protrudes beyond the skin layer at the wound edge, the cartilage should be carefully trimmed back so that the skin slightly overhangs it (Fig. 8-13).[45]

For extensive lacerations, a few stitches of 6-0 Vycril or Dexon can be placed in the perichondrium to bring together the underlying cartilage at important landmarks in the ear's architecture.

Skin sutures, however, and not the deep ties, are the mainstay of the repair of a cartilaginous laceration. The skin sutures are made such that the base of the suture loop passes through the perichondrium. Thus, the skin and cartilage are repaired simultaneously. Indeed, for small chondral lacerations this technique alone is sufficient, without the use of any buried ties.

Through-and-Through Ear Lacerations. In through-and-through lacerations of the ear, the

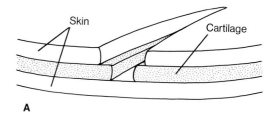

A

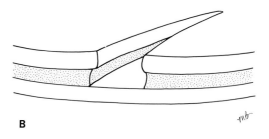

B

Figure 8-13 If the cartilage in the wound edge extends out further than the overlying skin (**A**) trim the cartilage such that the skin overhangs by about 1 mm (**B**).

perichondrium should be brought together with a few deep sutures of 5-0 or 6-0 Vycril or Dexon, as described in Wounds Involving the Cartilage, above. Following this, the skin on both sides of the ear is repaired with 6-0 polypropylene or nylon, with incorporation of the perichondrium in the suture loop. A running-type skin suture offers the advantage of increased ease of removal from the posterior aspect of the wound, which is important when one is trying to remove sutures without disturbing the configuration of the recently repaired cartilage.

Hematomas of the External Ear. A hematoma of the external ear can evolve into fibrous tissue which causes thickening and deformity of the ear. Therefore, acute external ear hematomas should be drained.

To drain a hematoma to the ear, the overlying skin is thoroughly cleaned and prepped. Then, after local anesthesia, a 3 to 4-mm skin incision is made at the most dependent portion of the hematoma, and the hematoma is evacuated. If the skin at the incision gapes open widely, a single 6-0 polypropylene suture can be placed; however, this is rarely needed. Some physicians place a small drain in the cavity left by the evacuated hematoma although we have not found this to always be necessary.

The wound is dressed with a circumferential compressive dressing (see Compressive Dressing, below). The pressure dressing is essential to retard reformation of the hematoma. The patient should return to the emergency department within 24 hours for a wound check, at which time the bandage is then replaced for an additional 3 to 4 days.

Auditory Canal Lacerations. Lacerations of the auditory canal are best treated by packing the canal with a nonadherent wick fashioned by wrapping Xeroform gauze around a tuft of cotton wool. The patient should be rechecked in 2 days, and a new wick placed for an additional 3 to 5 days. The wick tends to hold the lacerated edges in apposition and thus allows for healing to occur.

The ear canal generally does not require repair. An exception is when cartilage is exposed; such cartilage should be covered.

Lacerations with Tissue Loss. Tissue loss in ear lacerations is a major problem because the tightly adherent skin does not readily stretch to cover tissue defects. Skin grafting may be necessary.

Loss of both skin tissue and cartilage requires special techniques. Small defects (less than 0.5 cm), can often be closed primarily; however, a small ear will result. The closure is effected by excising small triangles in the antihelical fold as illustrated in Figure 8-14. These triangular wedges permit closure of the defect, without development of kinks within the natural curvature of the uninjured portion of the ear.

For larger defects, the authors generally recommend calling in a consultant. Remember that all recovered pieces of avulsed tissue should be cleansed and saved, as they may be used in the subsequent repair. However, even with microsurgical techniques, results are frequently disappointing.

Compressive Dressings. A pressure dressing to the ear is essential with all major ear injuries, including hematomas and lacerations involving cartilage. The posterior portion of the ear should be supported by a bolster made by wrapping gauze around moist cotton wool. A cast is then made of the anterior ear by wrapping Xeroform gauze around moist cotton wool and forming it to the ear. The entire dressing is then firmly secured down with a circumferential gauze wrap which goes all the way around the head (see Chapter 11).

The Nose

Anatomy

The nose is supplied by the infratrochlear nerve from above, which innervates the bridge

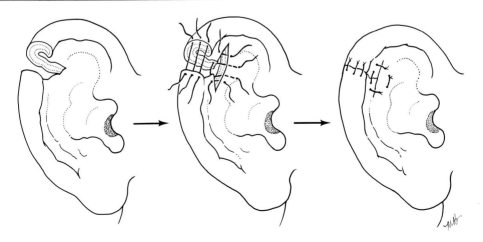

Figure 8-14 Ear wedge excisions to repair small tissue losses in the ear. The wedge excision is necessary to prevent buckling of the cartilage.

of the nose. The external nasal nerves on either side innervate the cartilaginous portion of the nose and the tip. The infraorbital nerve supplies innervation to the outer portion of the nose. The cartilage of the nose is not as tightly adherent to the skin as in the ear. The anterior septum of the nose is well nourished by an arterial plexus called Kesselbach's triangle. An injury to this plexus can lead not only to nosebleeds, but also to the formation of a septal hematoma.

Evaluation

The general appearance should be noted for obvious swelling or deformity. The leaking of clear water from the nares raises the concern of a cribiform plate fracture with a secondary cerebrospinal fluid (CSF) leak. Check for tissue loss, and preserve the tissue whenever possible.

The nasal bones at the bridge should be palpated for tenderness and instability. If a patient has crepitance of the nasal bones, a nasal fracture is diagnosed, even if the fracture cannot be discerned on nasal x-rays (which is sometimes the case).

The physician should inspect the nasal cavities, looking in particular for a septal hematoma. Septal deviation should also be noted. In addition, if a laceration is present, the nasal cavity should be checked to see whether the laceration is through-and-through. In the authors' experience, the otoscopes available in emergency departments are often inadequate to inspect the nose internally. A much better view of both turbinates and septum can be gained using a standard nasal speculum.

Extraocular muscles should be evaluated to check for a possible blowout of the orbital floor, which leads to an ipsilateral loss of upgaze.

As with other facial injuries, the maxilla should be pulled forward by exerting pressure with the thumb placed on the hard palate just behind the front incisors. Forward motion of the maxilla indicates a LeFort facial fracture.

Nasal bone radiographs are generally not clinically indicated. If there is deformity of the nose, or septum, the patient will require repair, even if radiographs fail to demonstrate the fracture. By contrast, if x-ray film shows a fracture but no discernible deformity of the nose or nasal

septum, no therapy is necessary. However, facial films can be useful to check for associated facial fractures.

Treatment

General. The skin of the nose is replete with sebaceous glands and tends to rip easily if the suture loop does not include some of the deep, fibrous layer. Inversion of the wound edges commonly occurs in lacerations involving the junction of the nares and the upper lip. However, this inversion can usually be prevented by placing the sutures quite close (about 2 mm) from the wound edge.

As with ear lacerations, no cartilage should be left uncovered by skin (or mucosa if the laceration extends to the inner surface), because otherwise chronic chondritis can result.

Sutures can be removed in 4 to 5 days for adults and 3 to 4 days for children. Skin tapes should be placed following suture removal. Because of the oily nature of the skin, paint the skin with tincture of benzoin before placing the tape strips, to increase adhesion.

Irregular Lacerations. Because of the lack of extra tissue in the nose, débridement should be kept to a minimum. Small skin sutures are used to tack the edges together. After healing has occurred, the patient can be referred for elective scar revision if needed.

Wounds Involving the Cartilage. As with the ear, when the nasal cartilage is lacerated or abraded it should be thoroughly cleansed by saline lavage, followed by direct preparation with dilute povidone-iodine solution. Debride only necrotic tissue. For extensive lacerations, a few stitches of 6-0 Vycril or Dexon can be placed to approximate the cartilage. However, also as with the ear, skin sutures, and not the deep ties, are the mainstay of the repair of a cartilaginous laceration. The skin sutures are made to pass through the perichondrium, and thus approximate skin and cartilage simultaneously.

As part of the aftercare, a small anterior pack consisting of Xeroform rolled over cotton to produce a small cylinder can be placed in the anterior nares to help support the injured cartilage. The pack need not be as extensive as those used to tamponade nosebleeds (see Chapter 11).

Through-and-Through Lacerations. The skin and cartilage are repaired as described above. In addition, a few ties of 5-0 Dexon or Vycril should be used to approximate the mucosal laceration, so that no cartilage is left open to the air. A small anterior pack is placed to support the injured cartilage (see Wounds Involving the Cartilage, above).

Lacerations with Tissue Loss. Whenever possible, the avulsed pieces of tissue should be recovered, cleansed with saline, and kept moist and cold. Small avulsions can be treated by reimplanting the defatted avulsed segment as a full-thickness skin graft. If the avulsed segment has been lost, or is too severely damaged to use, an ellipse of tissue can be taken from just above the clavicle or from behind the ear and used for grafting.

Large tissue defects are difficult to manage and are generally an indication for referral to the plastic surgeon.

Septal Hematoma. The physician should drain a hematoma of the nasal septum as soon as possible after the diagnosis is made. If these hematomas are left undrained, they become infected and necrose the nasal cartilage, leading to a permanent ''saddle nose'' deformity.

Septal hematomas are drained by making a small L-shaped incision at the most inferior portion of the hematoma (Fig. 8-15). The nose is then packed to prevent reaccumulation (special septal splints are also available) and the patient has a follow-up examination with a specialist in 24 to 48 hours.

THE UPPER EXTREMITY

The Hand

Anatomy

The hand is composed of two skin types. On the dorsal surface is loose skin without significant subdermal attachments. On the palm is thick skin which contains specialized septal attachments from the dermis to the fascia below. Injuries to the palm can lead to swelling on the dorsum of the hand, because the dorsal skin

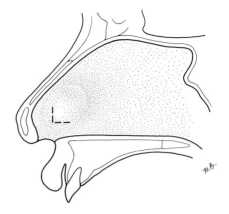

Figure 8-15 Draining a septal hematoma of the nose.

swells much more easily than the palmar skin. Treatment of hand lacerations differs on the dorsal and palmar surfaces.

The flexor tendons course through the volar surface of the hand from the forearm. The extensor tendons course through the dorsal surface. The tendons in the palm course through the deep palmar spaces and are surrounded by the bursae.

The metacarpal nerves divide into the digital nerves which then divide into dorsal and ventral branches.

In order to properly treat lacerations of the hand, the physician must have a good understanding of the anatomy of the hand. A detailed discussion of this subject is beyond the scope of this book.

Evaluation

Assess the sensation of the hand by checking for possible decreased two-point discrimination at the fingertips (radial and ulnar portions of the pad for each finger tested), as well as the routine examination for light touch and pinprick sensation on the remainder of the hand.

In lacerations of the dorsal aspect of the hand one must make a careful search for injury to the extensor tendons. If the patient experiences weakness or pain on stress testing of the extensor tendons, assume that a tendon laceration is present. Even superficial lacerations may involve the tendon because of the close proximity of the tendons to the surface.

Always beware of lacerations over the metacarpophalangeal (MCP) joints. These injuries frequently are the result of the patient striking another person's tooth. In about one-third of the cases, the patients do not report the true cause of the injury. Lacerations over the MCP joints should be considered to have penetrated the joint until either exploration, by enlarging the laceration to adequately visualize the full depth of the wound, or injection of the joint proves otherwise. The laceration may have been sustained with the joint flexed, and an injury to the capsule hence may not be visualized unless the joint is viewed in both the flexed and extended positions. Injection can be performed using sterile fluorescein dye, one drop per 5 cc sterile saline. This is then injected directly into the joint (entering opposite the side of the injury) and after 10 minutes the fluorescein escapes through a tear in the joint capsule and is readily seen when the wound is viewed with the aid of a Wood's lamp. If the joint has been penetrated the wound should not be closed; rather the patient should be referred to a consultant for open débridement and irrigation in the operating theater. Otherwise a severe, necrotizing infection from the flora of the saliva can result.

Lacerations of the volar surface of the hand pose a special problem in that there are many vital structures coursing through the palm. The area distal to the distal palar crease and proximal to the proximal interphalangeal joint is called "no man's land," because of the frequently poor functional outcome following injuries to this region. Therefore, lacerations that traverse the dermis must be fully evaluated for injury to the tendons, nerves, or arteries, and if present, should be repaired by a hand surgeon.

Just as with the extensor tendons, partial injury to the flexor tendons can be diagnosed by pain or weakness on stress testing. The deep and superficial flexors to the fingers should be checked as shown in Figure 8-16. The physician must remember that to check the superficial flexor to a finger, the action of the deep flexor must be negated by fixing the other digits in full extension. At times a tendon injury can be diagnosed even without stress testing. Complete or severe partial tendon lacerations can often be diagnosed by observation alone. Because of a

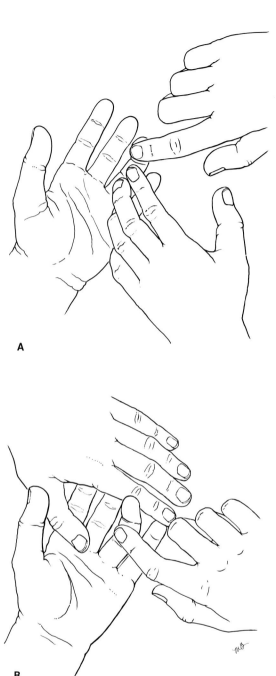

A

B

Figure 8-16 Testing the flexor tendons of the fingers. **A.** The flexor digitorum profundus is tested by resisting flexion of the distal phalanx while holding down the proximal and middle phalanges. **B.** The flexor digitorum superficialis is tested by resisting flexion of the middle phalanx, while holding the other fingers in full extension. With the other fingers in full extension, the flexor digitorum profundus is inactivated.

loss of balance between flexor and extensor tendons, when the hand is in the relaxed position a severed flexor tendon will result in one digit appearing in more extension than the others, as shown in Figure 8-17. The same phenomenon, though in reverse, occurs when an extensor tendon is severed.

Treatment

Control of Bleeding. In order to assess a wound, the bleeding must be under control. Bleeding should be controlled by direct pressure, or if necessary by placing a blood pressure cuff on the upper arm, elevating the arm to allow venous drainage, and then rapidly inflating the cuff to 250 to 300 torr, or about 100 mm above systolic pressure. First wrapping the upper arm with cast padding will make the pressure cuff more comfortable for the patient.

Bleeding should never be controlled by clamping blood vessels. The clamp will crush the artery, making future microsurgical anastomosis more difficult, and also can damage vital nerves that run in close proximity to the arteries.

Axiom: *Bleeding in the hand should not be controlled by clamping vessels. Rather, control the hemorrhage with direct pressure.*

Lacerations—General. Lacerations of the hand are divided into clean and contaminate injuries. A contaminated wound can be converted into a clean one by proper irrigation and débridement. The hand is one of the most infection-prone portions of the body, and as in all wounds, delays in suturing closed the wound increase the infection potential. Ideally, the physician should cleanse the wound as soon as possible after the patient is admitted into the emergency department. This task can be performed by ancillary personnel. The nature of the offending agent must also be considered. Knife wounds or those caused by glass fragments are generally clean, whereas wounds from industrial accidents and animal bites are not.

Clean wounds can be closed after irrigation with saline, and local antisepsis with dilute povidone-iodine prep solution (never use the cytotoxic detergent ''scrub''). Contaminated wounds should be repaired by delayed primary closure (see Chapter 7), and small lesions may be left to heal by secondary intent.

The skin should be closed with a nonpyogenic suture material such as polypropylene or nylon. As a general rule, no buried sutures are placed in the hand. Take care that the skin sutures do not pass so deeply as to pass through underlying tendons, nerves, or blood vessels.

The loose tissue of the dorsum of the hand often needs to be repaired using a vertical mattress stitch, to insure edge eversion.

The palm can be adequately repaired using simple sutures. However, because the palm has a special dermis which is adherent to the fascial sheath below, undermining should not be performed in the palm.

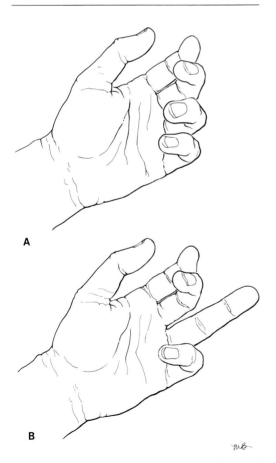

Figure 8-17 Severed flexor tendon leading to increased extension of the affected digit when the hand is in neutral position. **A.** The normal, relaxed hand. **B.** The effects of a severed flexor tendon of the fourth digit.

Repair of lacerations involving the web spaces can be facilitated by using a small, half-circle-shaped needle. (In most cases, the actual configuration of the needle is illustrated on the suture packet.)

In most cases the lacerated region should be splinted. The hand splint should be such that the fingers are in 20 degrees of flexion, and the MCP joints in 50 to 90 degrees flexion. Sutures can be removed at 7 to 10 days for lacerations not over a joint, and 10 to 14 days or more for areas over a joint.

Lacerations That Cross the Interphalangeal Joints on the Volar Surface. Remember always to evaluate the integrity of the joint capsule as well as the volar plate.

Generally speaking, these lacerations should be closed primarily rather than changing the orientation by a Z-plasty. In most patients there is excellent function following simple repair. Z-plasty may be performed on an elective basis in patients in whom contractures do develop.

U-Shaped Finger Lacerations. Shallow U-shaped lacerations of the fingers in which the U-shaped flap is small, and the base/length ratio less than 3:1, should be excised and allowed to granulate in. When these lesions are closed they can heal with elevation of the flap, and leave a permanently elevated deformity.

Lacerations of the Dorsal Hand with Atrophic Skin. In the elderly and in patients on chronic steroids, the skin over the dorsum of the hand is frequently paper thin. In such a case, a superficial laceration is best treated with skin-strips alone. If skin-strips alone are insufficient to close the defect, a gently performed horizontal mattress suture can be used, taking care not to pull too tightly, causing overlap of the edges. Simple sutures and vertical mattress sutures are not practical because they both tend to rip through the skin. Often grafting is necessary, which is best referred to a hand surgeon.

Tissue Loss. Wounds with more than a small defect may require grafting (except for fingertips, see Fingertip Amputations, below). If the wound is contaminated, the region should be cleaned and dressed, and the patient referred for grafting when there is less risk of infection.

If the laceration is clean, these wounds can be grafted using primary intent, with either a full- or a split-thickness skin graft. Most parts of the hand can be grafted using a full-thickness graft obtained from the inguinal region or the wrist crease. The antecubital region should not be used as a donor site because the scar is unpredictable.

Tissue Loss in the Palm. Tissue loss in the palm is perhaps one of the most difficult areas to deal with, because there is no ability to undermine the dermis, nor is there redundant tissue to pull from. Fortunately, this is not a common injury. These patients are probably best referred to a hand surgeon, because long-term treatment is often necessary. Initial therapy usually consists of a full-thickness skin graft and a firm hand dressing.

Tissue Loss over the Interphalangeal Joints. When there is full-thickness tissue loss over the interphalangeal or MCP joints with exposure of the extensor tendon, this must be covered. This can be accomplished with a split-thickness skin graft when simple apposition of the edges is not possible. The hand should be splinted.

Digital Degloving Injuries. This is often called a ring injury because the ring finger is the most commonly involved digit. The patient's ring hooks on to something during a fall, causing degloving of the skin. These patients should be referred to a hand surgeon.

If the degloving is partial, treatment consists of repositioning of the skin, elevating and immobilizing the hand, and administering systemic low-molecular-weight dextran. Some centers employ hyperbaric oxygen therapy. If the avulsion is complete, a pedicle flap can be attempted, but amputation is often necessary.

Fingertip Amputations. Fingertip amputations are common injuries that present to the emergency center. Depending on the amount of tissue loss and whether bone exposure has occurred, various regimes have been recommended. These include full-thickness and split-thickness skin grafts over the amputated portion, as well as rotation flaps for larger areas of tissue loss. For many years these techniques were not challenged. It was not recognized that if fingertip amputations are permitted to granulate in they will regenerate a new fingertip in a relatively short period of time. In numerous clinical studies, this conservative method of treatment yielded superior cosmetic and functional results compared to grafting or flaps. The fingertips that are allowed to granulate in have superior two-point discrimination on sensory examination, and tend to have better rounding out of the regenerated pad.[4,43,63,69,99,109,117,127,162]

Several systems to classify fingertip amputations have been devised. In perhaps the simplest system, a *type I* amputation involves only the distal flesh of the fingertip, and none of the nail bed. A *type II* injury involves the nail bed but none of the bone. A *type III* injury goes through both nail bed and bone, but is distal to the germinal matrix. A *type IV* injury goes through nail and bone, and involves the germinal matrix. As would be expected, the more distal injuries have the more favorable outcomes.

Therapy of fingertip avulsions in which there is either no bone involvement or the bone involvement is minimal consists of placing an occlusive dressing over the wound and changing this dressing at days 2, 4, 6, and 10. A splint should be employed to protect the fingertip during the healing process. In cases where bone is exposed and protruding at some distance from the tip, the exposed bone must be trimmed away with rongeurs. Hence, such cases are best referred to the hand surgeon.

Nail Bed Injuries. Certain basic principles should be followed concerning nail bed injuries.

1. There should be minimal débridement.
2. Remove the nail and accurately appose and repair the lacerated nail bed and root with 6–0 absorbable suture material. If the root cannot be repaired, refer the patient to a specialist.
3. The skin folds around the nail margin (the paronychium and the eponychium) must be preserved, and not allowed to form adhesions to the exposed nail bed when the nail has been removed. Adhesions can be prevented by replacing the nail (after cleansing) as a stent, or by packing the fold

with a nonadherent dressing such as Xeroform gauze.

Immediate primary reconstruction of the nail bed and root is the treatment of choice. Before a discussion of the methods of repairing the various injuries of the nail bed, the anatomy and generation of the nail must be understood. The nail matrix is formed from three sites: the nail bed, the roof matrix in the eponychial region, and the root matrix. The most important areas to be preserved for the generation of a normal nail are the roof and root matrices. In a child, if the nail bed is destroyed, a normal nail will usually eventually regrow. However, if the nail root and roof matrix are destroyed, an entirely normal nail will never grow back. Thus injuries that seem to obliterate the nail itself (nail bed injury) frequently heal well, whereas smaller lesions at the base (root and roof matrix region), in which the greater portion of the nail initially appears normal, can eventually yield a gnarled, unsightly nail.

Figure 8-18 illustrates the repair of a nail bed laceration that does not involve the paronychial or eponychial skin folds. The nail has been removed to facilitate repair and then replaced as a stent to avoid adhesions at the folds.

Figure 8-19 illustrates a laceration that includes the paronychial skin fold. The nail bed is repaired in the usual fashion, then a single suture of Prolene or nylon is used to repair the

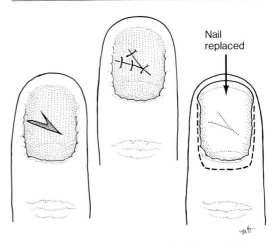

Figure 8-18 Repair of nail bed laceration. The nail has been replaced as a stent.

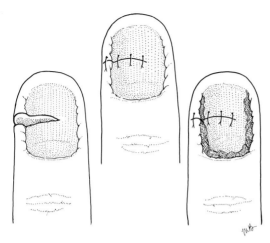

Figure 8-19 Repair of laceration involving nail bed and paronychial skin.

skin. This skin suture should be just deep enough to repair the dermis, but not so deep as to include the nail bed below. Since the nail has been too badly damaged to serve as a stent, the nail folds are packed with Xeroform gauze.

Figure 8-20 illustrates the use of a mattress stitch to replace avulsed nail bed matrix tissue into its proper position following an injury. The matrix must be placed back into position, or new nail growth will not occur.

The stent—either the cleansed native nail or the Xeroform gauze—should be left in place for approximately 1 week. The finger should be splinted and covered with a normal wound dressing. A wound check at 2 days is advisable. Skin

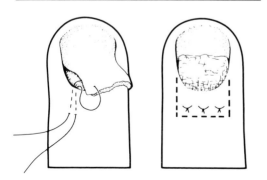

Figure 8-20 Replacement of a nail bed that has become avulsed. *Source:* Reprinted from *Procedures and Techniques in Emergency Medicine* (p 317) by RR Simon and BE Brenner with permission of the Williams & Wilkins Company, Baltimore, © 1982.

stitches can be removed in 7 to 10 days. The nail bed stitches are left to resorb. The patient should be advised that while the chances for forming a new nail are good when the injury is not severe, there is no guarantee as to what the final outcome will be.

In cases where the distal tuft is fractured, in addition to the nail bed laceration, the patient is given parenteral cephalosporin or nafcillin in the emergency department, followed by oral antibiotics, since it is an open fracture. However, distal tuft osteomyelitis following open fracture is fortunately not common.

Subungual hematoma. When a subungual hematoma is larger than 3 to 4 mm in diameter, it can be drained by either drilling through the nail (a 19-gauge needle can be used to bore through the nail) or by burning a hole with a hot paperclip.

An extensive subungual hematoma is almost always associated with a nail bed laceration. We feel that the nail should be removed (in the case of a large hematoma, the nail will eventually fall off anyway) and the laceration repaired. The nail is then replaced as an anatomic stent. If one does not repair the nail bed, a step-off ridge may occur.

Extensor Tendon Lacerations. Extensor tendon injuries heal with fewer complications than flexor injuries because the extensor tendons do not have tendon sheaths.

A partial laceration to an extensor tendon generally heals well without sutures to the tendon. The affected region is splinted in a position midway between full relaxation and contraction. The tendon will heal in 3 to 6 weeks. After the first 2 weeks the physician should remove the splint and the patient should start to perform passive extension exercises. This prevents contractures. Active motion, however, should not be initiated until the fourth week.

Although a complete extensor tendon laceration can be repaired by the emergency medicine specialist, such cases are still best referred to the specialist who will be responsible for long-term followup, including rehabilitation. Of the numerous techniques for suturing tendons, we prefer the simple figure-eight stitch as shown in Figure 8-21.

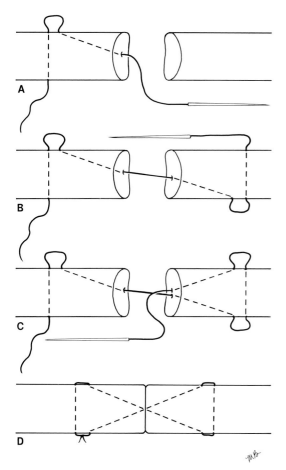

Figure 8-21 Extensor tendon repair using a figure-eight stitch.

Flexor Tendon Lacerations. Because of the presence of the tendon sheath over flexor tendons, there is a higher complication rate than for extensor tendon tears. In flexor tendons, adhesions can develop between sheath and tendon. Therefore we recommend that patients with flexor tendon lacerations be referred to a consultant.

Foreign Bodies in the Hand (see also Chapter 9, Section Foreign Bodies). Glass, metal, and wood are the most common foreign materials seen in hand wounds. While some particles are inert and cause little reaction, others can cause significant problems. Most glass fragments are radio-opaque. Anteroposterior, lateral, as well as oblique radiographs should be taken, because the glass is extremely hard to spot if it is overlying a bone.

Small glass fragments may not require removal. The patient should always be informed that some small glass fragments may be retained, and that the body will form a barrier around these. Larger fragments frequently cause symptoms if left in place, and should be removed if possible. Sometimes the physician must wait until a fibrous capsule forms about the foreign body before finding and removing the object.

Metallic particles may remain inert and asymptomatic and thus not require removal. Particles of metal that subsequently become symptomatic should be removed at a later date.

Wood particles are usually radiolucent, and hence invisible on x-ray examination. Some wood particles have been stained with toxic agents such as aniline, resins, or oils that can induce a marked inflammatory response if the wood splinter is not removed.

Simple Crush Injuries. Crush injuries to the hand are common in industry. The deep tissue is often congested and poorly perfused, while the surface skin appears relatively healthy. Therefore repeated examinations of the hand on an outpatient basis for less severe injuries and on an inpatient basis for severe injuries are necessary.

Mangled Hand Injuries. Treatment of these injuries in the emergency department is difficult. Only a cursory assessment of the circulation and gross neurologic assessment should be done, as well as preliminary films. Open wounds should not be probed because this may increase the risks for infection. Parenteral antibiotics should be given early. The hand should be cleansed, covered with sterile dressings, and immobilized pending arrival of the consultant. Immediate surgery is needed when external hemorrhage cannot be controlled (except with an inflated blood pressure cuff), or when rapid, progressive swelling threatens to compromise the vascular supply. Blind clamping of vessels should never be performed, as is true for all hand injuries.

Some surgeons feel that hyperbaric oxygen therapy can limit the amount of necrosis following a severe crush injury.

Injection Injuries. High-pressure injection injuries from paint guns and grease guns cause extensive dissection of the noxious substances into the deep tissue planes of the hand. In some instances, the pressure equals 15,000 pounds per square inch. Frequently the physician can be fooled by the benign appearance of the small entry site. These patients must be referred for immediate débridement in the operating room. Films should be obtained because many of the materials are radio-opaque (such as leaded paints).

Gas injected under pressure may dissect widely and penetrate the systemic circulation, causing circulatory collapse.

Injection with water under pressure can frequently be treated by admission for observation, without operative débridement.

Injection of liquid may spread widely and block nerve conduction, delaying the onset of pain and further deluding the examiner into thinking that he or she is dealing with a trivial injury. The patient later complains of a sudden feeling of hotness in the hand. As mentioned already, when dealing with a toxic substance, fasciotomy and open débridement is necessary.

The Wrist, Forearm, and Elbow

Anatomy

Whenever a laceration of the forearm is seen the physician must institute a careful search for penetration of the fascial layer lying just deep to the dermis. In the volar wrist, for example, course the median and ulnar nerves and arteries, and the flexor tendons of the hand, all within a space of some 5 to 6 cm (Fig. 8-22).

Injuries to the dorsum of the wrist threaten the extensor tendons of the wrist, thumb, and fingers, as shown in Figure 8-23.

More proximally, in the forearm itself, the structures most commonly injured are the flexor and extensor muscles supplying the hand; however, damage to nerves and arteries should still be ascertained. Elbow injuries threaten the major veins, nerves, and arteries on the volar side, and the olecranon bursae on the extensor side, as well as causing concern that injury may extend into the joint capsule itself (Fig. 8-24).

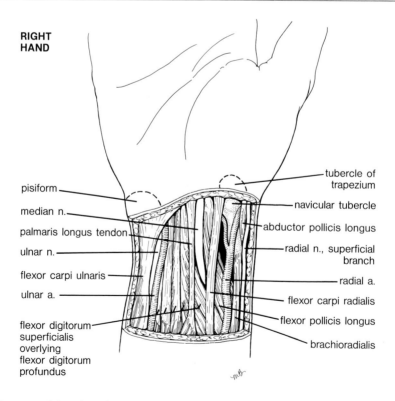

Figure 8-22 Structures of the wrist, volar aspect.

RIGHT HAND

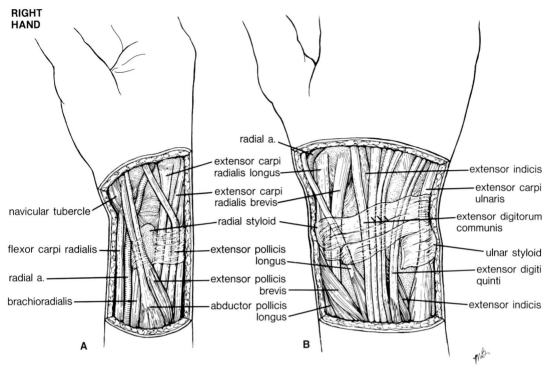

navicular tubercle

flexor carpi radialis

radial a.

brachioradialis

radial a.

extensor carpi radialis longus

extensor carpi radialis brevis

radial styloid

extensor pollicis longus

extensor pollicis brevis

abductor pollicis longus

extensor indicis

extensor carpi ulnaris

extensor digitorum communis

ulnar styloid

extensor digiti quinti

extensor indicis

A   **B**

Figure 8-23 Structures of the wrist, radial (**A**) and dorsal (**B**) aspects.

RIGHT ARM

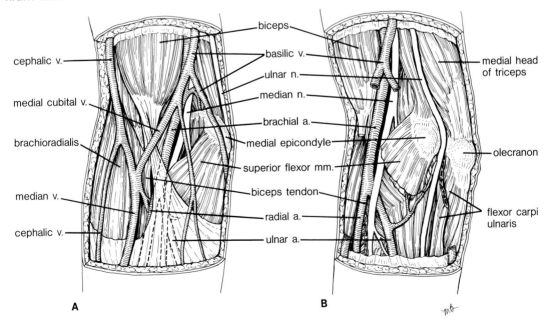

cephalic v.

medial cubital v.

brachioradialis

median v.

cephalic v.

biceps

basilic v.

ulnar n.

median n.

brachial a.

medial epicondyle

superior flexor mm.

biceps tendon

radial a.

ulnar a.

medial head of triceps

olecranon

flexor carpi ulnaris

A   **B**

Figure 8-24 Structures of the antecubital fossa (**A**) and medial aspect of the elbow (**B**).

Evaluation

A laceration deep to the fascial layers should be carefully evaluated for tendon, muscle, or nerve involvement, as well as a possible arterial laceration. A normal sensory motor examination should be performed, including a check for two-point discrimination at the fingertips. The evaluation of the deep and superficial finger flexors is discussed in The Hand, above.

When a nerve lesion is suspected the patient has either complete sensory or motor loss distal to the lesion, or subjective paresthesias.

Allen's test demonstrates loss of flow through either the radial or ulnar artery. To perform the test, first have the patient clench the fist, and then apply sufficient pressure over the radial and ulnar arteries to occlude blood flow. After approximately 1 minute, the patient relaxes the hand and the pressure is released over the ulnar artery. The hand should promptly blush pink. The test is then repeated, this time checking for flow through the radial artery. Allen's test is important because a spurious pulse may be detected in a completely severed artery, owing to a transmitted proximal pressure wave and spasm distally.

Multiple lacerations over the wrist and forearm most commonly occur secondary to suicide attempts, and proper psychiatric evaluation should be made.

Treatment

General. As with the hand, care should be taken that the suture loop of the skin suture does not inadvertently incorporate any of the deep nerves, arteries, veins, or tendons. Except to repair deep rents in muscle fascia, deep sutures are to be discouraged due to the increased risk of infection.

Whenever possible, use the natural skin creases (such as the flexor creases of the wrist) as landmarks to guide the repair. Skin sutures can be 4–0 or 5–0 nylon or polypropylene. Sutures over extensor surfaces should be left in place 7 to 14 days and be followed by skin tape; sutures in nonmoving regions or flexor surfaces can be removed in 7 days. The extremity should be splinted if the laceration is over a region of motion.

Lacerations of the forearm that are macerated or have major tissue loss can usually be closed by excisional débridement, undermining, and approximation of the edges. In the forearm and elbow there is ample tissue for such therapy. Even large defects can usually be repaired using a vertical mattress suture.

Lacerations with Injury to Nerves, Arteries, Muscles, and Tendons. All lacerations to major arteries require prompt referral for microsurgical reanastomosis.

If there is complete injury to tendon, muscle, or nerve there will be complete loss of function. All complete injuries should be referred for repair in the operating room. If a partial injury of a tendon or muscle is suspected, and the functional impairment is minimal, the physician may perform closure of the wound by primary intent in the emergency department. The extremity should then be splinted. If a large partial injury is suspected the patient should be referred.

Lacerations of the Posterior Elbow (Olecranon Bursa Injuries). Lacerations of the posterior aspect of the elbow may involve the olecranon bursa. In addition, the ulnar nerve courses lateral to the medial epicondyle and its function should be checked.

Lacerations involving the ulnar nerve should be referred to a specialist. Lacerations of the olecranon bursa that are clean and of the shear type (as in a knife-induced laceration), should be irrigated with copious saline, prepared with dilute povidone-iodine solution, and closed with skin tapes. Shallow skin sutures may be used in place of skin tape if care is taken not to go down to the bursa with the suture loop. A suture that passes into the bursa can lead to a chronic draining sinus track which can be extremely difficult to manage. The physician should apply a pressure dressing, followed by a dorsal splint which holds the elbow at 90 degrees of flexion. A wound check should be done after 48 hours. The splint can be removed after 4 to 5 days, and the sutures taken out after 2 weeks.

Macerated lacerations over the olecranon bursa commonly follow motorcycle injuries in which the patient scrapes the elbow along the ground. In these wounds it is frequently difficult to distinguish where the bursa begins and the dermis ends. The wound should be irrigated with copious normal saline under high pressure (see Chapter 4). Debride all soiled and nonviable tissue, even if some of the bursa needs to be removed. The wound is then bandaged and a posterior splint is applied to the arm. The patient returns in 3 to 4 days for delayed primary closure (see Chapter 7). The redundant tissue around the elbow offers excellent opportunity to excise and close these lesions.

For all bursal injuries, caution the patient that a sinus track may develop. In addition, there is the possibility of inflammatory or septic bursitis.

Lacerations over the Antecubital Fossa. Lacerations over the anecubital fossa must be carefully examined for damage to the deep structures. On the medial aspect lie the brachial artery and the median nerve (Fig. 8-24). Always check for damage to these structures. The radial and ulnar nerves are in a deeper, more protected region, and are therefore less frequently involved. Whenever an expanding or pulsatile hematoma is noted, consider the possibility of brachial artery injury. Arteriography may be needed to confirm the injury. The biceps tendon rarely is involved in lacerations over the antecubital region. Patients who suffer damage to antecubital nerves, arteries, or tendons should be referred to a specialist for possible operative repair.

Upper Arm and Axilla

Anatomy

In the upper arm are located the major flexor and extersor muscles of the arm. The brachial artery and the median nerve are located in the groove that is formed between the biceps and triceps muscles.

The axilla houses a host of important structures in a small area. These structures include the brachial plexus, the axillary artery, and a number of peripheral nerves.

Evaluation and Treatment

The physician should insure that a full neurovascular examination of the upper extremity is performed. Upper arm lacerations can be directly explored for damage to deep structures. The physician should avoid deep sutures, which should only be used to close rents in muscle fascia. The skin should be closed with either 4–0 or 5–0 nylon or Prolene. The arm should be immobilized in a sling for 5 to 7 days for large lacerations. Sutures can be removed after 7 to 10 days.

Axillary lacerations pose a special problem because of the numerous deep structures. Lacerations that extend deep to the subcutaneous tissue and involve the deep fascia must be considered to have injured these structures until proven otherwise. Neurovascular examination should include a check of the blood pressure in both arms. Auscultation with the stethoscope and possibly a Doppler device should be done to check for bruits. Decreased blood pressure in the affected arm or the presence of a bruit is an indication for arteriography. The physician should refer any laceration that does involve the nerves or arteries in the axilla to the attention of a specialist.

THE LOWER EXTREMITY

The Foot

Anatomy

The dorsal skin is usually pliable and is closely applied to the underlying extensor tendons. The sole of the foot possesses a specialized skin area with a thick cornified layer, and a dermis that has specialized septal and fibrous attachments to the underlying fascial layer.

Evaluation

The physician should carefully evaluate lacerations to the dorsum for extensor tendon damage. In lacerations to the sole, a soft tissue film should be obtained if there is a question of a retained foreign body such as a piece of glass or metal fragment. Also for lacerations of the sole, carefully check for any injury to the flexor tendons.

Always suspect bone involvement whenever a wound is painful on movement of the foot. This is especially true with puncture wounds.

The patient should be questioned about diabetes, because the sensory impairments in this disease make foot lacerations more common and also severely impair healing.

Treatment

General. Foot lacerations pose special problems in laceration repair similar to hand injuries. Lacerations to the sole are difficult to debride because the adjacent tissue does not slide over easily to cover a defect. In lacerations of the dorsum, the thin skin tends to invert, thus the vertical mattress suture is often indicated.

Lacerations to the Dorsum of the Foot. If a partial extensor tendon laceration is present, but there is no obvious functional impairment, then the skin alone should be closed without placing a suture to repair the tendon. This is because a deposit of fibrous tissue often forms around sutures placed to repair tendon lacerations, possibly due to the constant stress on the area caused from the pressure of shoes.

Lacerations to the Sole of the Foot. Débridement of lacerations to the sole should be very minimal if at all. These wounds should be carefully irrigated and cleansed. No subcutaneous sutures should be placed and the wound edges should be brought together without undue tension. The skin sutures must pass deep enough to include the fibrous dermis, because sutures that are entirely within the cornified epidermis tend to rip out. Silk sutures are more comfortable to the patient to walk on but carry a higher infection potential. Therefore nylon or polypropylene sutures are preferable. A foam shoe insert makes walking more comfortable. When possible, the foot should be kept elevated for the first 2 days following the repair.

When the flexor tendons are damaged, repair should probably take place in the operating room or be performed by a consultant. It is difficult to treat damage to this region in the emergency department.

Lacerations between the Toes. Lacerations between the toes should be repaired with a half-circle needle. These lacerations rarely involve the metatarsal nerve or other deep structures.

Puncture Wounds to the Sole (see Chapter 9). Puncture wounds to the foot from clean objects (e.g., a sewing needle, an unused nail) should be cleansed with saline externally, and dressed with a Band-Aid.

Punctures caused by contaminated objects (such as a rusty nail) or those that first puncture the shoe and sock (and therefore have the potential for impaling small amounts of material deep within the wound) should be treated by excising a rim of about 2 mm of skin in a circumferential manner around the puncture site. The physician should attempt to remove possible foreign materials, using a fine-tipped splinter forceps. Then the wound should be irrigated, holding the tip of the catheter about ¼ cm above the puncture site. The physician should apply a clean bandage, and ideally the patient should keep the foot elevated for approximately 48 hours.

Patients with foot punctures should be educated about the possibility of a late bone infection, which would become evident by causing pain in the foot commencing days to weeks following the initial injury.

Foreign Bodies in the Sole (see Chapter 9). Glass foreign bodies in the sole can at times be brought to the surface simply by injecting locally with an anesthetic solution. A needle is used to infiltrate the tissue around the entry site with about 3 cc, or until there is noticeable edema. The increased hydrostatic pressure (which is especially great owing to the fibrous nature of the sole) may cause the glass to poke to the surface.

The Lower Leg

The skin of the lower leg often is atrophic, particularly in the elderly and patients on steroid therapy. There is little subcutaneous support, especially over the tibia, and this makes repair difficult. Sutures placed in the skin commonly pull through (see Chapter 7). The technique for suturing a laceration in atrophic skin is shown in Figure 8-25. Alternatively, small wounds in the region can be repaired with skin strips. Extensive lacerations may require advancement flaps or grafting and may require referral to a specialist.

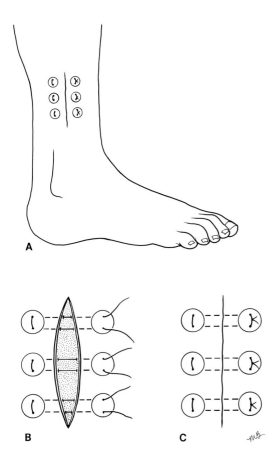

A

B   **C**

Figure 8-25 Suturing lower leg lacerations in patients with atrophic skin.

Lacerations of the lower leg otherwise can be treated similar to the technique described for forearm lacerations.

The Knee

Anatomy

Lacerations of the knee must be evaluated for extension into a number of important structures. Anteriorly, the prepatellar bursa lies just beneath the skin over the patella (Fig. 8-26). Lateral lacerations near the fibula may involve the peroneal nerve. Posterior laceration may involve the popliteal artery and the tibial nerve (Fig. 8-27). Any laceration can enter into the joint space.

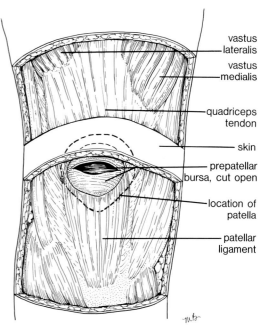

vastus lateralis
vastus medialis
quadriceps tendon
skin
prepatellar bursa, cut open
location of patella
patellar ligament

Figure 8-26 The anterior aspect of the knee. See text for discussion.

Evaluation

Any laceration in which one cannot be certain of intra-articular extension should be examined for joint involvement. A large laceration into the joint capsule can be detected by aseptically placing a needle or angiocath into the joint and infusing sterile saline (use bacteriostatic solution for injection). The saline will leak out of the defect in the capsule. Placing a few drops of sterile methylene blue into the saline will aid in detection of extravasation. To detect a small penetration, place a drop of sterile fluorescein into 50 cc of sterile saline and infiltrate into the joint. An elastic wrap is then placed around the knee for 10 minutes. Then the wrap is removed and a Wood's lamp used to detect extravasation of the dye out from the joint.

Treatment

Lacerations of the knee over the extensor surface should be repaired using a vertical mattress stitch. This yields a stronger, more protective repair against the force of the flexing knee.

RIGHT LEG

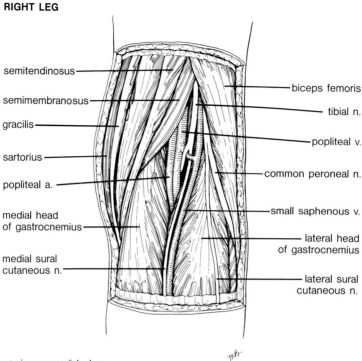

semitendinosus

semimembranosus

gracilis

sartorius

popliteal a.

medial head
of gastrocnemius

medial sural
cutaneous n.

biceps femoris

tibial n.

popliteal v.

common peroneal n.

small saphenous v.

lateral head
of gastrocnemius

lateral sural
cutaneous n.

Figure 8-27 The posterior aspect of the knee.

Tissue loss over the extensor or flexor surface of the knee is generally easily repaired by first undermining and then approximating the skin edges.

Abrasions with ground-in dirt should be scrupulously cleansed of all foreign material, otherwise a permanent tattoo can result.

After repairing a moderate or severe laceration, splint the knee at 20 to 30 degrees flexion with a posterior splint. Sutures can be removed at 7 to 10 days for posterior lacerations, and 8 to 14 days for anterior lacerations.

THE TRUNK

The Chest, Back, and Abdomen

Laceration to the chest, trunk, and abdomen generally do not pose special problems, and can be repaired with simple skin sutures of 4–0 or 5–0 nylon or polypropylene. Sutures should be left in place for approximately 1 week.

The Perineal Region

Anatomy

The skin of the penis is thin with little subcutaneous fat. Deep to the skin lie the corpus cavernosum dorsally on either side, and the corporus spongiosum ventrally in the midline. The testicle is covered by the tense, tough, fibrous outer coat called the tunica albuginea. This layer is difficult to penetrate but must be checked in any lacerations of the scrotum.

The female external genitalia consist of the labia majora, which are covered with skin, and the labia minor, covered with a mucosal epithelium.

Evaluation

Always assume that lacerations to the penis or scrotum involve deep structures, unless proven otherwise. If the deep structures are involved, urologic consultation should be obtained.

Genital or perianal lacerations in children should always alert the physician to possible child abuse. External lacerations are often accompanied by more severe injuries to the rectal or vaginal mucosas. Spasm of the anal sphincter is a sign that the sphincter has been damaged.

Treatment

Lacerations to the penis or scrotum that involve only the skin layer can be closed with simple sutures. Avoid deep sutures as there is little subcutaneous tissue and it is easy to penetrate the vital structures deep to the skin. When a laceration is deeper and involves the testical or deep structures in the penis, urologic referral is indicated.

Lacerations of the vagina usually do not require repair if they are small, longitudinal, and the deep muscular tissue is intact. If the laceration is deep, repair can be accomplished using a speculum and an instrument tie with a long needle holder. An absorbable suture such as 4–0 Dexon or Vycril can be employed. The muscle layer can first be closed with a running deep suture, beginning at the proximal, and ending at the deep extent of the wound. The same suture can then be used to close the mucosa, using running simple sutures. A laceration over the skin between the anus and the vagina can be closed with a subcuticular stitch. Always be certain that no suture is allowed to pierce through the rectal mucosa, because a chronic sinus tract infection can result.

The physician can close perianal lacerations with a single layer of fine nylon or polypropylene, again taking extreme care that the suture loop does not pierce the rectal mucosa.

Chapter 9

Bites, Punctures, and Foreign Bodies

ANIMAL BITES

This section discusses animal bites, particularly those from mammals, including dogs, cats, rats, and humans. The first part of the section deals with bites in general. The second part of the section discusses the individual animal species.

General

Infection Potential of Animal Bites

Saliva from the mouths of animals contains scores of different bacteria, including aerobes and anaerobes, both gram-negative and gram-positive types. Fungi can also be cultured from the crevices between the teeth.

Some confusion arises about the bacteriology of animal bites because the frequency with which a given microbe is cultured from an animal's saliva is not the same as the frequency with which that same microbe is cultured from an infected wound caused by a bite of the animal. Similarly, the frequency with which a given microve is cultured from fresh bite wounds (and therefore contains the saliva of the animal) is not the same as the frequency with which the microbe is cultured from wounds that subsequently become infected. In choosing antibiotics to treat an infected bite, the physician should be guided by the types of organisms that are commonly cultured from infected bites rather than by the types of organisms that are cultured from the animals' mouths.

Local Therapy of Animal Bites

Animal bites constitute contaminated wounds, and therefore should be treated with high-pressure saline irrigation (see Chapter 4). We recommend using a 35-cc syringe fitted with an 18- or 19-gauge needle or plastic catheter, holding the tip of the catheter 3 to 4 mm above the skin surface.

Following irrigation, about 2 mm of tissue should be trimmed from the wound edges, using either a scalpel or sharp iris scissor.[194] Following débridement, the wound may require repeat irrigation to remove tissue fragments.

Following irrigation and débridement a 1 percent povidone-iodine solution (i.e., a 1:10 dilution of the 10 percent stock solution; do not use the detergent scrub) should be directly applied to the open wound.

Small puncture wounds caused by animal bites should likewise be treated with excision of a thin rim of skin from the wound edge (see Puncture Wounds, below), but should not be sutured closed.

With dog bite lacerations, following proper irrigation and débridement, the infection rate in wounds sutured closed primarily appears to be essentially the same as in wounds that are left open.[18,194] Extrapolating to other animals, bite lacerations in well-perfused areas, such as the face, can be sutured closed primarily, keeping the number of deep stitches to a minimum.

If the wound can be repaired using skin tape, this technique is particularly attractive because of the lower incidence of infection following closure with tape compared to skin sutures.[52]

For infection-prone areas, such as the hands, the authors recommend either skin tape or repair by delayed primary closure (see Chapter 7, section Delayed Primary Closure).

For abrasions and superficial lacerations, treatment should consist of irrigation followed by application of topical povidone-iodine solution.

If the decision is made to give prophylactic antibiotics, the first dose should be given immediately in the emergency department. In laboratory experiments prophylactic antibiotics are not effective beyond 3 hours after wounding.[52] Recommendations for prophylactic antibiotics for specific animal bites are presented later in this chapter.

Infected Bites

Patients frequently seek help only after the animal bite has become infected.

Patients who present with signs and symptoms of infection within the first 24 hours following the bite most often are infected with *Pasteurella multocida*.[70] *P. multocida* can be cultured from the mouths of cats, dogs, horses, hens, cows, ducks, rabbits, pigs, and even veterinary students. Of patients with culture-proven *P. multocida* infections, one-fifth have a dark yellow or serosanguinous discharge, one-third have regional adenopathy (frequently painful), and one-fourth are febrile.[70] The most common cause is cat bite or cat scratch.

Patients infected with other organisms, such as *Staphylococcus aureus* and hemolytic and nonhemolytic streptococci, typically develop symptoms more than 24 hours after the bite.

If an eschar covers the infected wound, it should be unroofed. Pus can be Gram's-stained and sent for culture. The wound should then be irrigated with copious saline and a 2-mm rim of tissue should be excised from the wound edge, as described above in Local Therapy of Animal Bites. The wound should be covered with a clean, absorbent dressing and allowed to heal by secondary intent. If the bite is to an extremity, the extremity should be splinted for the first 3 to 5 days, and kept elevated. Crutches are recommended for lower extremity bite infections.

The choice of antibiotics for bite infections is discussed below in the section on individual animal bites. We recommend giving the first antibiotic dose parenterally if there is local cellulitis, adenopathy, or systemic signs. Patients who appear systemically ill (high fever or white count) generally require admission to the hospital. Others can be discharged on oral antibiotics, with a return follow-up in 24 to 48 hours.

Rabies[122,171]

Several species of mammals in the United States harbor the rabies virus.

Bats. The virus is endemic in bats, because in bats infection with rabies does not always progress to the fatal illness seen in humans. Bats can pass the virus directly to humans via bites. In addition, spelunkers exploring bat-infested caves have contracted the virus through contact with the animals' secretions. Bats also pose a threat by biting domestic animals, including cattle.

Wild Carnivores and Scavengers. Rabies virus has been cultured from the brains of many wild scavengers and carnivores. The most common of these are:

- Bat
- Coyote
- Wild dog
- Fox
- Mountain lion
- Raccoon
- Skunk
- Wolf

Domestic Animals. In 1984, the most commonly rabid domestic animal in California was the cow.[171]

Domestic dogs and cats rarely harbor rabies, although there have been exceptions. The offending animal should be quarantined for approximately 14 days, and killed and examined for rabies virus if it shows a decline in behavior.

Animals immunized for rabies can still become infected with the wild virus and spread the disease to humans.

Stray dogs are responsible for only about 1 to 2 percent of dog bites in urban areas.[174] The physician should contact the local department of health to determine whether or not to give rabies vaccine to a person bitten by a stray animal.

Rodents and Lagomorphs. Rodents (mice, rats, squirrels, and chipmunks, but excluding bats), and lagomorphs (rabbits) pose little threat. These animals rarely harbor rabies virus.[139] In addition, most species produce little saliva and thus have decreased potential for spreading the virus even if rabid. Prophylaxis is rarely indicated for rodent or lagomorph bites, but the emergency physician should be guided by the most current recommendations of the local health department or the Centers for Disease Control (CDC) in Atlanta.

Rabies Prophylaxis. Local health departments and the CDC perform yearly surveys of the presence of rabies virus in both domestic and wild animals. Therefore, the emergency physician should be informed of the most current recommendations as to which animal bites will require rabies prophylaxis.

On the initial visit, the patient should be given both the first in a series of human diploid cell vaccine injections and, in addition, human rabies immune globulin (RIG). Some physicians administer half of the RIG dose as a local infiltration at the site of the animal bite. The immune globulin should not be given at the same site as the vaccine. The patient then must return at regular intervals to complete the five shots in the series of the vaccine.

Public Health Report. Most states require that all animal bites be reported to the local department of health.

Specific Animal Bites

Dog Bites

Epidemiology. Dogs account for more animal bites than all other species combined.[174] Large mixed breeds and German shepherds account for nearly one-third of all bites.[120] The attack rate by German shepherds is nearly twice what can be accounted for by the prevalence of the breed in the community.[120] On the other end of the spectrum, Labrador retrievers, although common, rarely attack people.[120]

In adults the extremities are most commonly bitten, while in children it is the face.

Infection Potential. Hand wounds become infected more commonly than wounds to other regions, and puncture wounds become infected more commonly than lacerations.[18] Overall, about 5 percent of dog bites become infected.[2] Despite the traditional doctrine to the contrary, suturing only seems to raise the infection rate by a single percentage point.[18] In fact, in one study in children in which the treatment protocol included high-pressure irrigation, wound edge excision, and prophylactic antibiotics, the overall infection rate was only 0.5 percent per wound, less than the rate for elective surgical procedures at the same hospital.[194]

Multiple organisms can be cultured from the saliva of a dog's mouth, including *P. multocida*, gram-positive cocci, gram-negative rods, and anaerobes. As mentioned in Infection Potential of Animal Bites, above, the bacteria present in fresh, uninfected dog bites differ significantly from the bacteria in infected wounds. In one study, by far the most common organisms cultured from infected dog bites were *S. aureus* and *Staphylococcus epidermidis*.[80] *P. multocida* and Enterobacter were the next most common causative organisms. The incidence of *P. multocida* in infected wounds (25 percent) approximately equaled its incidence in fresh, uninfected wounds (32 percent). *S. aureus*, however, which could be cultured from only one-fourth of the fresh wounds, accounted for half of the wound infections.

Prophylactic Antibiotics. Several studies have investigated the efficacy of prophylactic antibiotics in preventing wound infections following dog bites.[25,26,57,80,155] Several studies have shown a trend for an improved outcome with antibiotics. For example, Rosen, in a study of 66 wounds, found an overall infection rate of 6.7 percent in the group given either dicloxacillin or erythromycin, compared to 11 percent in those given placebo; and an infection rate in hand wounds of 12 percent in the antibiotic group compared to 30 percent in the control population.[155] However, none of these differences proved to be significant. In an excellent report, Brown and Ashton pointed out that none of the studies that have currently been published on dog bites have large enough sample sizes to document a benefit from antibiotics, assuming that such a benefit exists.[18]

Until the question of whether or not to give prophylactic antibiotics for dog bites is settled, the authors favor the use of antibiotics for infection-prone wounds, such as puncture wounds and wounds to the hands. The authors recommend that either a first-generation cephalosporin such as cephalexin (Keflex) or a penicillinase-resistant penicillin such as dicloxacillin be given for 4 days following the injury, and that the first dose be administered in the emergency department as soon as possible. Although penicillin is the drug of choice in treating *P. multocida*, it is a poor agent against *S. aureus*, and *S. aureus* causes more infections in dog bites than *P. multocida*.

Treatment of Wound Infections. The wound should be irrigated and debrided in the usual manner (see Infected Bites, above). Pus can be sent for Gram stain and culture. Sutures must be removed.

Patients who develop infections within 24 hours of the animal bite should receive penicillin to guard against *P. multocida*, possibly with the addition of an antistaphylococcal agent as well, such as a first-generation cephalosporin or a semisynthetic penicillin. Tetracycline should be administered to penicillin-allergic patients who are over 8 years of age. Erythromycin has poor activity against *P. multocida*. Keflex and dicloxacillin have intermediate activity against *P. multocida*.

For patients who develop infections later than 24 hours after the bite, treatment should be with either Keflex or dicloxacillin, possibly with the addition of penicillin to cover for *P. multocida* infection (although *P. multocida* infection rarely develops more than 24 hours following the bite).

The authors favor giving the first dose of antibiotics parenterally in the emergency depart-

ment. Patients who appear toxic need to be admitted for continued parenteral therapy.

Cat Bites

Infection Potential. Unlike dog bites, which usually cause lacerations, cat bites result in multiple puncture wounds which leads to a greater potential for infection. The majority of cats harbor *P. multocida* in their mouths, and, in contrast to dog bites, *P. multocida* is the most common cause of infection following cat bites and scratches.[55]

Prophylactic Antibiotics. The question of whether or not to administer prophylactic antibiotics for cat bites has been studied much less extensively than for dog bites. However, in one study, oxacillin, 500 mg qid for 5 days following the cat bite, led to a significantly lower incidence of infection than the placebo group.[56] We recommend prophylaxis for cat bites with either penicillin, dicloxacillin, or oxacillin. Penicillin-allergic patients over 8 years of age can be treated with a course of tetracycline. Erythromycin is not effective against *P. multocida*.

Treatment of Wound Infections. The wound should be irrigated and debrided in the usual manner, and pus sent for Gram's stain and culture (see the sections Infected Bites, above, and Puncture Wounds, below). Even with appropriate antibiotic care, the infection does not resolve if there is undrained pus.

Penicillin should be administered, possibly with the addition of an antistaphylococcal antibiotic such as dicloxacillin or Keflex. The authors favor giving the first dose of antibiotics parenterally. Patients who appear toxic need to be admitted for continued parenteral therapy.

Human Bites

Patterns of Injury. Human bites frequently do not pierce the skin, and thus result only in local ecchymosis. More vicious assaults often result in the avulsion of tissue. One particularly important type of human bite is on the hand, typically over one of the metacarpophalangeal joints, incurred when an individual strikes another person's mouth (see Chapter 8).

Patients with human bites frequently delay in seeking help, and once in the emergency department, often fabricate a story to explain the injury.

Infection Potential. The human mouth contains several pathogens that can lead to severe, necrotizing infections. In one study of infected human bites to the hand, 7 percent of patients eventually required an amputation.[160]

A common pathogen in infected human bites is *Eikenella corrodens*, a facultative anaerobic gram-negative rod. The organism takes between 3 and 11 days to grow in culture medium.[161] Penicillin is the drug of choice for *E. corrodens*. The organism is also sensitive to cephalothin (Keflin) but resistant to methicillin.[161]

Prophylactic Antibiotics. We recommend prophylactic antibiotics for human bites, although their efficacy has yet to be proven. Penicillin provides excellent coverage for oral pathogens. Erythromycin can be used for penicillin-allergic patients.

Treatment of Wound Infections. Patients with infected human bites to the hand require admission and parenteral antibiotics. If the bite enters the joint space, operative débridement is required as well. Purulent material should be sent for Gram's stain and aerobic and anaerobic cultures. Antibiotic coverage should include penicillin, plus an antistaphylococcal agent such as a cephalosporin or a semisynthetic penicillin.

Rat Bites

Incidence. Rat bites usually occur in the domestic setting. Commonly the bites occur at night, to exposed portions of the body (such as the face).

Infection Potential and Antibiotic Prophylaxis. In a study of 50 rat bites treated solely with irrigation and minimal débridement, only one wound infection occurred.[139] Bacteria cultured from fresh wound sites were usually sensitive to both Keflex and dicloxacillin. However, because of the low incidence of infection, prophylactic antibiotics are not necessary.

Treatment of Wound Infections. Infected rat bites should be treated with cephalexin (Keflex) or dicloxacillin.

Lion and Tiger Bites

Like their domestic cousins, large cats carry *P. multocida* in their mouths. However, the deep penetration of the fangs leads to more serious sequelae, such as *P. multocida* meningitis.[22]

Fish Bites

Wounds following fish bites, or more commonly cuts in workers who handle fish and other meats can develop an indolent cellulitis called *"fish baiter's" disease*. The infection typically consists of a slow-spreading (1 cm/day) cellulitis, affecting one of the digits. The causative organism is Erysipelothrix, a small gram-positive rod. Penicillin is the treatment of choice.

Seal Bites

Wounds contaminated with seal saliva (or possibly infectious material from seal pelts) can lead to an unusual condition known as *seal finger*. The affected finger swells dramatically secondary to a predominantly lymphocytic infiltrate. The disease responds to tetracycline, but the causative organism has not yet been identified.

Great White Sharks

The bacteriology of the mouth of the great white shark has recently been elucidated.[21] The giant carnivore harbors numerous marine bacteria, including vibrio species. Any one of a number of antibiotics (including gentamicin, cefoxitin, tetracycline, and chloramphenicol) is adequate to provide coverage against the bacteria cultured from the shark's mouth.

Lacerations in Meat Packers

There is anecdotal evidence that lacerations caused by knives used in cutting meat may have an increased infection rate.

PUNCTURE WOUNDS

General

Puncture wounds carry a higher infection potential than lacerations. This is evident from the fact that dog bites that result in puncture wounds result in infections significantly more frequently than those that result in skin lacerations (see Dog Bites, above). These infections most likely result from the introduction of pathogens and particles of debris into the deep tissue. An eschar of serous fluid or blood rapidly forms at the top of the puncture site, trapping the foreign material below. Even if the patient presents to the physician before an eschar has formed, the small entry wound makes irrigation of the deep portions of the wound nearly impossible.

Puncture wounds result in both soft tissue and bone infections.

The most common soft tissue infections are cellulitis and microabscesses. The patient usually presents with pain and local redness 24 to 48 hours after the injury. Septic arthritis can occur if a joint capsule is pierced (see section Hand in Chapter 8).

Patients with bone infections usually present 5 days or more after the injury complaining of local pain, and in some cases malaise and fever. The most common site for osteomyelitis following a puncture wound is the foot. Interestingly, the most common pathogen causing osteomyelitis of the foot following a puncture wound is *Pseudomonas aeruginosa*.[82,96,111,118,147] These infections usually involve cartilaginous parts of the bone, such as the articular surface or the growth plate.

Treatment

Clean Puncture Wounds

For relatively uncontaminated puncture wounds, such as occur when the skin is pierced by a clean nail, the only therapy is to irrigate the injured site with normal saline and apply a topical antiseptic such as povidone-iodine solution. As with all wounds, the physician should make sure the patient's tetanus injections are up to date. The puncture site should be gently probed. If superficial, the injured area should be covered with a Band-Aid for approximately 3 days and the patient educated about the signs of infection. For foot puncture wounds, if the wound goes deep enough to involve a bone or joint, the patient should use crutches and the affected foot should not bear weight for 4 days. Elevation is also advised.

Contaminated Puncture Wounds

Our experience has been that if a dirty puncture wound (as from a rusty nail or a cat fang) is treated by excising a small plug of tissue at the puncture site, followed by vigorous irrigation, the incidence of wound infection is decreased. The rationale for this therapy is twofold: a larger puncture site is more amenable to irrigation; and a larger puncture site seals over less rapidly, allowing the deep tissue to drain.

The easiest way to enlarge the puncture wound is to anesthetize the skin, and then, using a no. 11 scalpel blade and forceps, excise a 2 to 3-mm-wide full-thickness rim of skin around the puncture site, as illustrated in Figure 9-1.

Alternatively, a 4-mm disposable skin biopsy punch can be used. The deep tissues are not excised, because it is generally not possible to ascertain the path of the wound beneath the surface. The site is next irrigated under pressure

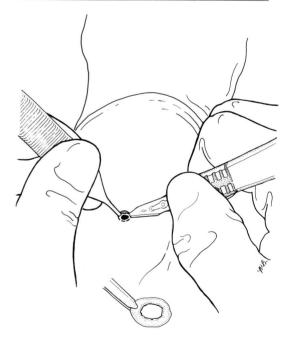

Figure 9-1 Treatment of a contaminated puncture site. The top of the illustration shows the excision of a 2mm rim of tissue using a No. 11 blade. At the bottom of the illustration is a close-up of the excised tissue.

with normal saline, using a 35-cc syringe fitted with an 18-gauge angiocath. The stream is directed directly over the puncture site, with the tip of the catheter approximately 0.5 to 1 cm above the wound. Placing the catheter tip directly within the wound cavity may cause ballooning of the deep tissues with saline, and for this reason is not recommended. Finally, 1 percent povidone-iodine solution is applied directly to the wound, using a moistened, sterile gauze, and then the wound is covered with a sterile dressing.

The patient is advised to keep the injured region elevated for the first 48 hours, and to return to the emergency department if there are any signs of infection.

For foot punctures, the wound should be probed. If the wound is deep enough to involve bone or joint, the patient should not bear weight for 4 days. A follow-up visit in 7 days is advised.

Early Infection

In many cases patients first present after the puncture wound has become secondarily infected. As already mentioned, the most common early infections are cellulitis and microabscess.

Therapy consists of excising a skin plug around the puncture site (see Contaminated Puncture Wounds, above). For infections that are more than trivial, the affected region can be splinted for 3 to 4 days. For foot punctures, supply the patient with crutches and advise no weight bearing until the infection has cleared.

If systemic signs and symptoms are present, the first dose(s) of antibiotics should be parenteral. Other infections can be adequately treated with oral antibiotics for 7 to 10 days. For patients with systemic signs and symptoms, the choice of antibiotics can be guided by wound Gram's stain and culture. Cultures are not usually needed for patients without systemic symptoms.

A patient who develops septic arthritis following a puncture should be referred to an orthopedist for drainage, followed by admission to hospital for administration of parenteral antibiotics.

Late Infection (Osteomyelitis)

Patients who develop bone infections after a puncture wound usually present with pain in the affected region, usually 5 days or more after the initial injury. The evaluation should include a complete blood count, sedimentation rate, and x-ray films to look for periosteal reaction. If the film is normal but the sedimentation rate is elevated, or if the physical examination is suggestive, we recommend a bone scan of the affected area. Especially in the case of the foot, these infections can progress to the point of partial limb loss. Therefore the patient should be referred to a specialist for definitive therapy, which often will include open débridement of the affected bone, sending samples for Gram's stain and culture. For osteomyelitis of the foot following a puncture wound, initial antibiotic therapy should provide pseudomonal coverage.

FOREIGN BODIES

General

Imbedded foreign bodies are a frequent problem presenting to the emergency department. The most common areas of the body affected are the forehead (following a car accident in which the forehead shatters the windshield), the eye, the hand, and the foot.

Evaluation

Suspicion of a foreign body is raised by the mechanism of injury. Whenever broken glass leads to a laceration, look for retained fragments. With puncture wounds on the sole of the foot, consider the possibility that the patient stepped on a pin which subsequently broke, leaving a fragment imbedded in the foot. A wound infection that fails to heal following appropriate antibacterial therapy should raise the question of a retained foreign body.

On physical examination, manipulation away from the puncture site frequently causes pain secondary to movement of the foreign body deep to the skin. After appropriate topical anesthesia, probing the wound track with a 25-gauge needle (or a long 22-gauge needle for deeper wounds) is often fruitful in evaluating for foreign material.

Axiom: Never probe for an imbedded foreign body until the region has been adequately anesthetized.

A probing needle can often detect imbedded foreign material, especially metal or glass. If the needle strikes a piece of glass, a distinctive grating sensation is felt by the examiner, and at times the scratch of the needle against glass can be heard. Similarly, metal fragments are easily detected when touched by a probing needle. Wooden objects, especially hardwood splinters, can usually be detected by the probing needle.

Even if the probe of the wound with a needle is negative, the region still should be subjected to x-ray examination. X-ray films help confirm the diagnosis of a retained foreign body. A soft tissue anteroposterior and lateral view of the affected area should be undertaken, as well as an oblique view is there is underlying bone. The oblique view increases the chances of getting a clear film of the foreign body without the picture being obscured by underlying bone.

Metallic foreign bodies show up easily on x-ray film. In addition, recent studies have shown that in excess of 90 percent of glass shards (not just leaded glass, as has been previously taught) show up on the x-ray film.[177] Wooden and plastic objects pose more of a problem, because these objects frequently blend imperceptibly with the surrounding soft tissues.

Shallow foreign bodies can usually be removed without much trouble, using either a smooth forceps, a foreign-body forceps, or a small hemostat. Frequently it is necessary to make an incision in the overlying skin wide enough to allow the tip of the instrument to fit beneath the surface.

For deeper objects, consider placing two needles into the skin at right angles over the entry site, or taping bent paperclips over the entry site prior to sending the patient for x-rays. The metallic object serves as a stereotactic guide for the removal of the foreign body, as shown in Figures 9-2 and 9-3.

Even if the methods described above are used, the search for small foreign bodies is often futile.

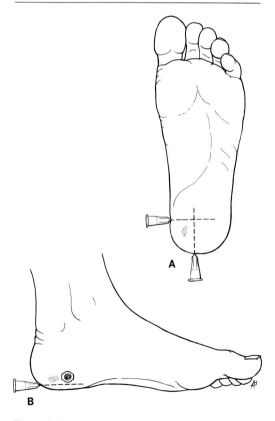

Figure 9-2 Inserting two needles at right angles to one another prior to taking x-ray film can serve as a stereotactic guide for removal of foreign bodies. Note that the two needles are inserted at different depths, to aid in localizing the object. **A.** View looking down on the heel. **B.** Side view.

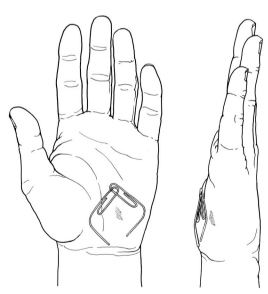

Figure 9-3 Taping two interlinked paperclips over the presumed location of the foreign object prior to taking x-ray film helps localize the foreign body. This technique, although not as precise as the two-needle technique (see Fig. 9-2), avoids puncturing the skin.

We recommend that before attempting the removal of the object, the physician advise the patient that such attempts, especially in regard to glass foreign objects, often fail. If the object cannot be located and removed following a reasonable effort, the region should be dressed and the patient referred to a surgeon to have the object removed at a later date. With time, a foreign body reaction causes collagen to be deposited around the object. This fibrous shell makes the object easier to locate when the patient returns for elective removal at 3 to 4 weeks.

Thorns, cactus spines, and wooden splinters should be removed with a gentle twisting motion. Otherwise small barbs tend to catch on the skin as the object is removed.

Chapter 10

Burns and Abrasions

THERMAL BURNS

First-Degree Burns

General

In *first-degree burns* the skin appears erythematous and is tender to the touch. Sensation and perfusion are intact. There is no blistering of the skin, but peeling of the epidermis usually occurs within 7 days of the injury.

Common causes of first-degree burns are minor scald injuries and sunburn.

Treatment

In first-degree burns, the integument is intact, hence secondary infections are rare, and there is no desiccation of the dermis and no eschar formation.

Therapy consists of analgesics and cautioning the patient not to traumatize the injured skin. Wound dressings and salves are not necessary.

Second-Degree Burns

General

In *second-degree burns* there is blister formation as fluid from the injured area pools beneath the epidermis. In superficial second-degree burns, sensation is intact (beneath the blister) and the capillary fill is normal. In deep second-degree burns, involving necrosis of the superficial dermis, there may be impairment of both cutaneous sensation and perfusion.

Deep second-degree burns have the potential of converting to full-thickness (third-degree) burns if injured dermal vessels, which were initially patent, subsequently thrombose. Wound infection frequently causes conversion of a partial-thickness to a full-thickness injury.

Therapy

Patients with extensive second-degree burns (greater than 20 percent of the body surface area), as well as significant burns involving the hands, feet, perianal region, or genitalia should be referred to a burn center for admission. The wounds should not be dressed with antibiotic creams prior to transfer, as the overlying creams will make it harder for the receiving surgeons to differentiate between full- and partial-thickness burns.

The resuscitation of the victim of a major burn is not within the scope of this book.

Small second-degree burns in which the roof of the blister is intact are ideally treated with a bulky, protective wrap (such as Kerlex) to prevent the blister from breaking. Prior to wrapping, physician should gently cleanse the wound. The patient should return for frequent follow-up visits.

Healing beneath an intact blister occurs more rapidly than when the blister is unroofed, presumably because there is no desiccation of the top dermal layer, and the new epidermal cells do not have to migrate beneath an overlying eschar. The blister roof also serves as a barrier against infection.

In patients in whom the blister subsequently breaks (as well as in those who present with open wounds), the dead skin can be easily debrided off using a thumb forceps and an iris scissor. The area is irrigated with saline. Then the open wound is treated with an antibiotic ointment or cream, such as silver sulfadiazine or bacitracin, and a dressing placed. The patient then requires daily dressing changes. With each dressing change the old antibiotic cream should be completely removed and new cream applied.

Some practitioners treat all second-degree burns with a 3-day course of penicillin to prevent a secondary infection with beta-hemolytic streptococcus. This practice has been questioned, however. In a recent study, the overall infection rate in second degree burns was 3 to 4 percent with or without prophylactic antibiotics.[13]

Third-Degree Burns (Full Thickness)

General

Full-thickness burns are injuries that destroy both the epidermis, dermis, and the epidermal cells in hair follicles and glands within the dermis. The burned area can appear white or bronze. The skin feels leathery, and there is loss of cutaneous sensation and perfusion.

Healing is by granulation from viable skin at the periphery of the wound. The thick eschar peels off in a period of 1 week or more.

Therapy

Patients with extensive third-degree burns (greater than 10 percent body surface area) and third-degree burns involving the hands, feet, perianal region, or genitalia should be referred to a burn center for admission.

The definitive therapy for third-degree burns is skin grafting. We recommend early referral for grafting (1 to 2 days after the initial injury) in order to decrease the total period of disability as well as the risks of secondary infection.

ELECTRICAL BURNS

Low-Voltage Injuries

Low-voltage burns, such as occur from standard house current, are usually simple thermal injuries caused by the electrical arc. Although systemic sequelae (such as cardiac arrhythmias) can occur, there is no charring of the deep tissues as occurs with high-tension electrical burns. Local therapy is the same as listed above for thermal injuries.

High-Voltage (High-Tension) Injuries

High-tension electrical cables can carry current measuring in the thousands of volts. The high-voltage current often incinerates deep tissues within its path. Thus a patient may present with trivial-appearing surface entry and exit burns, but may have complete necrosis of the muscles and nerves that were in the path of the current.

These patients generally require immediate transfer to a burn treatment center.

ABRASIONS (SEE ALSO CHAPTER 11)

An *abrasion* is an injury in which the outer skin layer is scraped away. With superficial abrasions only the upper, cornified epidermis is removed. There is little or no bleeding and regeneration is prompt. With deeper abrasions there is loss of the epidermis and dermis, exposing the underlying dermis to infection and desiccation. The risk of infection and delayed healing is naturally much greater than with the more superficial injuries. Regeneration must come from the epidermal cells in the epidermal appendages such as sweat glands and hair follicles.

With full-thickness abrasions, the entire depth of skin is lost. Healing is from normal tissue at the periphery of the wound.

Interestingly, abrasions tend to heal more promptly and with a lower incidence of infection than burns of equal depth. Whereas pseudomonal infections are common with burns, the same is not true for abrasions. This difference probably stems from the fact that in abrasions, the underlying tissues are relatively uninjured whereas in burns there is thermal damage to the tissues beneath the level of frank necrosis.[104]

Evaluation

As with any injury, the sensory-motor status and the perfusion of the affected area should be assessed. For minor abrasions, it is sufficient if the patient had an injection of tetanus toxoid within the past 10 years. For deep abrasions, the last tetanus booster should have been administered within the past 5 years.

Cleansing of the abrasion is important for two reasons. First, irrigation flushes away overlying bacteria that could infect the area. Second, irrigation helps remove particulate matter imbedded in the wound, which, if not removed, will lead to accidental tattooing of the skin.

If irrigation alone does not remove all foreign material, the abrasion must be scrubbed with either a sterile surgical brush or a gauze sponge soaked in saline. Never cleanse or scrub abrasions with detergent-containing solutions, or with prepackaged scrub-brushes with an attached sponge that contains povidone-iodine *detergent*. The detergent (and not the povidone-iodine solution) causes severe damage to any exposed dermal cells (see Chapter 4).

After the wound has been properly cleansed and debrided, all that is left is to apply the dressing. The epidermis serves two functions: it keeps bacteria from invading the dermis, and it protects the dermis from desiccation. The purpose of the dressing, therefore. is to provide these functions until the epidermis has regenerated. An antibiotic ointment both protects the dermis from superficial necrosis (due to desiccation), and, to some degree, retards infection. The authors prefer bacitracin ointment, because it is inexpensive, available without prescription, and seems to induce fewer allergic reactions than the ointments that contain neomycin.

The patient should be instructed to reapply the ointment each day and then cover the wound with a standard bandage.

Instead of a topical ointment, the abrasion can be equally well protected with any one of several occlusive dressings, such as polyurethane film (Op-Site, Biocclusive). These occlusive bandages should be removed every 2 to 3 days to check for any signs of infection, and a new bandage placed. Considering that the bandages must be changed, the total cost for the occlusive dressings usually exceeds the cost for topical ointment.

Chapter 11

Aftercare

This chapter deals with wound aftercare and is applicable to most of the classes of injuries discussed in this book. The first part of this chapter deals with various aspects of wound aftercare. We also discuss discharge medications, discharge instructions, wound checks, suture removal, and scar revision. The second part of the chapter takes a more detailed look at the effects of wound dressings on wound healing. Some of these effects are surprisingly marked. The last part of the chapter deals with the actual mechanics of bandaging, including choice of materials, general bandaging techniques, and finally bandaging by body region.

GENERAL WOUND AFTERCARE TOPICS

Dressing the Wound

After a wound has been repaired, the surrounding skin should be cleansed of any remaining blood or iodine. In some cases it is reasonable to document that the motor examination is still intact, especially if suturing has been in the region of tendons. Sensation, however, will be abnormal due to the lingering effects of anesthesia. The wound should be covered with an appropriate dressing.

Prior to the formation of the epithelial layer, lacerations are susceptible to infection from bacterial pathogens. With time, however, the wound becomes increasingly resistant to contamination. In a classic experiment, guinea pigs were subjected to abdominal lacerations down to and including the muscular layer.[44] The wounds were then sutured, and at various time intervals from the time of injury the wounds were swabbed with a fresh suspension of *Staphylococcus aureus*. The animals were then observed for the development of wound infection. The results are presented in Table 11-1.

Table 11-1 Infection Rates in Sutured Lacerations Contaminated with *Staphylococcus aureus* at Varying Amounts of Time from Closure.

Wound Age When Contaminated	Infection Rate (%)	Infection to Muscle
0 hr	100	Yes
2 hr	100	Yes
6 hr	100	No
12 hr	83	No
24 hr	66	No
48 hr	56	No
72 hr	36	No
4 days	10	No
5, 6, 7 days	0	No

Source: Surgery, Gynecology & Obstetrics (1933;56:762), Copyright © 1933, Franklin H Martin Memorial Foundation.

Protection from contamination is needed during the first 3 to 4 days following the injury. Wounds need to be covered early on to prevent wound infection, but what type of dressing is best?

Occlusive dressings, as opposed to nonocclusive bandages, appear to speed the healing process and improve the cosmetic appearance of the wound. A full discussion of the experimental effects of different types of bandages and ointments on wound healing appears in Effects of Bandages and Topical Agents on Wound Healing, below.

Discharge Medications

Outpatient Antibiotics

The *preoperative* administration of antibiotics has a definite and experimentally documented role in decreasing the incidence of wound infections in elective surgical procedures. However, in experimental studies, if such therapy is delayed more than 3 hours after the procedure, the benefit is lost.[49,115] For accidental wounds, therefore, the common practice of giving a patient a prescription to fill for an oral antibiotic should not be effective in decreasing the incidence of infection. The delay to therapy is too great. Indeed, several studies investigating the use of oral antibiotics for lacerations have shown them to be of no benefit in decreasing the infection rate.[87,92,148,191]

Clean, shear lacerations do not require antibiotic prophylaxis, since the infection rate with proper wound toilet is low. Antibiotics may be indicated for infection-prone injuries such as impact (crush) lacerations and certain animal bites, but therapy should be started as soon as possible after the patient presents to the emergency department. Vigorous cleansing of the wound seems to increase the time period after the injury during which antibiotics are still effective, but to quote Edlich and colleagues: "When the decision is made to initiate a preventive antibiotic regimen, the drug(s) should be administered immediately."[52] For infection-prone wounds the authors advocate the early administration of an appropriate antibiotic in the emergency depart-

ment, followed by the outpatient administration of the same antibiotic for 4 days after the injury.

Analgesics

Pain is frequently an unpleasant part of the recuperative period following any injury. The pain is usually greatest during the first 24 hours and then subsides. Pain is less in patients treated with occlusive bandages compared with those treated with gauze dressings.[186] The reappearance of pain 2 or more days following the injury should make the practitioner suspect a wound infection. A muscle injury with late spasm also causes increasing pain, however, there are no local signs of infection. Because the development of pain after 2 days can be a danger sign, analgesics should be limited to the immediate postinjury period and should not be overly potent. For a simple laceration, plain acetaminophen or acetaminophen with codeine should suffice. For extensive abrasions and burns, more potent analgesics, such as oxycodone, may be needed for the first 24 to 36 hours.

Ointments

Protective bandages cannot be applied to all parts of the body. Therefore, in regions such as the lips and the eyelids, where bandaging is impractical, application of an ointment every 3 to 4 hours can serve as a substitute. We recommend bacitracin, Neosporin, or Silvadene. The first two agents are available over the counter in most states, and are much less expensive. The neomycin in Neosporin can be sensitizing in some patients.[145]

The effects of ointments on wound healing is discussed more extensively in Effects of Bandages and Topical Agents on Wound Healing, below.

Bandages

For the initial bandaging in the emergency department, a nonadherent layer should be placed first, to facilitate subsequent removal of the wrap. Polyurethane film (Op-Site, Tegaderm, Insure IV, and Biocclusive) and foam (Epi-Lock) dressings, and hydrocolloid dressings (Dvoderm), range in price from $1.00 to $3.00.[186]

Medicated (Xeroform, Betadine) and nonmedicated (Adaptic, Vaseline gauze, Vigilon) moist dressings range in price from $0.85 to $3.00 for equivalent size bandages.[186] Nonadherent dry dressings (Telfa, Burn Dressing, Dermacell, Owens, Micron) range in price from $0.20 to $4.00.[186] Special biologic dressings (Mediskin, Biobrane, and Hydron) can range from $20 to $37.[186] The authors have found the less expensive dressings perfectly suitable for most applications. (See also Effects of Bandages and Topical Agents on Wound Healing, below).

The number of bandaging products available over the counter is staggering. The physician can assist the patient by recommending the most reasonably priced product that is best suited for the specific injury. Simple Band-Aids are economical and quite adequate for most small wounds.

Vitamins

A good balanced diet should insure proper healing for the average patient. However, patients on corticosteroids benefit from topical vitamin A (1,000 U/g cream) during the healing period. An oral supplement (25,000 U/day) is also effective, but the systemic use of vitamin A can also reverse the effects of the steroid on a systemic level, with possible adverse affects (such as in renal transplant patients with rejection). Vitamin A increases the rate of epithelialization in patients on chronic corticosteroids but does not restore normal wound contraction.[106]

Sunscreens

Sunscreens should be used for 3 to 6 months for sun-exposed wounds and surrounding skin, to avoid differential pigmentation of the healed region. Patients can begin use of the sunscreen after healing has taken place, that is, about 2 weeks following the injury. The authors recommend a sunscreen with a rating of 8 or greater.

Discharge Instructions

Dressing Change

Especially when numerous dressing changes are needed, such as for a perirectal abscess, the physician should instruct the patient and family about how to rebandage the wound. Such instruction can often be done by emergency department orderlies or technicians.

Elevation

For the first few days following the injury, elevation of the wounded region will decrease edema. Edema is especially damaging in sutured lacerations, because of increased tension of the tissue within the suture loop. The authors recommend that patients be instructed to keep affected extremities propped up for at least the first 48 hours. In the case of facial lacerations, patients should attempt to sleep with the head elevated on two pillows.

Immobilization

Immobilization is a key part of wound aftercare, particularly for extremity wounds. Simple finger splints can be used for the fingers. Well-padded posterior splints are adequate for knee, ankle, and elbow injuries. Palm injuries are best immobilized in a bulk dressing (see Figure 11-19).

Hot or Cold Packs

During the first 2 days following a burn, laceration, or abrasion, the ideal temperature for wound healing is body temperature. Excessive heat disrupts growth of the epithelial layer, while subnormal temperatures delay epithelialization.[121] Note, however, that ice is an ideal early treatment to counteract the edema of soft tissue contusions and sprains.

Keeping the Wound Dry

One of the usual instructions for patients with fresh lacerations is to keep the wound dry. As it turns out, however, brief periods of moisture do not harm healing of head and neck wounds. In a study of 200 such injuries half the patients were instructed to keep the wound dry, and the other half were allowed to briefly wash the injured region with soap and water beginning the day after the injury.[79] The wounded region was redressed immediately after washing. No differences could be discerned between the two groups.

The authors recommend that patients with head and neck lacerations be allowed to briefly wash the injured area with plain water, avoiding soap which has been shown irritating to wounds.[16] The injury should then be promptly re-dressed.

Instructions for Patients Admitted to the Hospital

The emergency physician should provide the specific aftercare instructions both to the patient and to the admitting physician.

Work Disability

Duration of disability, of course, varies with the nature of the injury. The emergency physician should provide a written, 24-hour excuse from work. Lengthier excuses should be provided by the industrial or follow-up physician.

In instances where the extremity must remain splinted for a prolonged period (e.g., following a tendon injury or a laceration over the extensor surface of a joint), this should be indicated on the disability form.

Wound Check

Signs of wound suppuration and cellulitis usually appear after 48 hours with simple lacerations, burns, and abrasions. Animal bites are an exception, frequently showing signs of infection within 24 hours of the injury. Hence, for an infection-prone wound the patient should be instructed to return for an examination of the wound 2 days following the injury, and perhaps sooner with bites. Infection-prone wounds include abrasions in which there was ground-in foreign material, any wound in which there was a moderate delay before emergency department treatment, underlying host disability such as diabetes mellitus, and most bites.

In the case of non-infection-prone wounds, the patient still should be instructed to look for

signs of infection, and to return if any of these signs are present.

Wound checks are also indicated in cases of lacerations with borderline perfusion at the wound edge (such as flap lacerations), and in cases involving a nerve, artery, or tendon injury in a patient initially difficult to assess due to anxiety or intoxication.

When a patient returns for a wound check, the bandages should be removed. The neurovascular status should be assessed. Wounds should be "rolled" with a sterile applicator to check for expressible pus, as shown in Figure 11-1.

In wounds that are 3 to 4 days old, 4 mm of erythema at the rim of a laceration probably represents normal neovascularization and should not be confused with cellulitis, which causes a wider rim of erythema, and is usually tender.

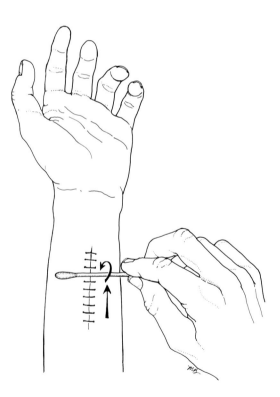

Figure 11-1 Rolling the wound with a sterile applicator often expresses purulent fluid if an infection is present. A small amount of serous fluid is not indicative of an infection.

Complications

Nerve Damage Not Noticed at Initial Evaluation

With lacerations nerve fibers become severed. No repair is possible for small fibers. If, however, the distribution of anesthesia follows the distribution of a major peripheral nerve, such as the digital nerve in the hand or the median and ulnar nerves in the wrist, the patient should be referred to a surgeon for possible repair. Peripheral motor nerves, such as the facial nerve, also require microsurgical repair. Peripheral nerves can still be repaired 2 weeks or more following an injury, and thus generally no damage results from the deficit being missed during initial examination.

Tendon Damage Not Noted at Initial Evaluation

Tendon damage not initially noted at the time of suturing frequently will be picked up either at the time of wound check or suture removal. The tendons can still be repaired; in fact, some surgeons routinely delay definitive repairs for 2 weeks postinjury. Hence appropriate referrals should be made.

Wound Infections

Five to 10 percent of wounds sutured in emergency departments become infected. The rate of infection following burns and abrasions varies with the extent of the injury.

Therapy of wound infections is as follows:

1. Possible minor infection (increased erythema and tenderness at the wound edge, but the patient is afebrile, there is little or no pus, and no fever, lymphyangitis, or regional adenitis). With this clinical picture the differential is between early infection and neovascularization. For lacerations, consider removing every other suture and placing tape strips in the gaps. The authors recommend beginning antibiotic therapy with either a semisynthetic penicillin such as dicloxacillin (250 mg qid for 7 to 10 days) or a first-generation cephalosporin such as cepha-

lexin (500 mg qid for 7 to 10 days). The patient should return for a follow-up check in 2 days.

In cases where there is scant purulence, without cellulitis or induration, suture removal and irrigation are all that is required.

2. Intermediate infections (obvious cellulitis, lymphangitis, lymphadenitis, often with low-grade fever). For lacerations, remove sutures, irrigate away pus, and allow the wound to heal by secondary intent. For burns and abrasions, unroof the eschar if pus is present, and irrigate. (For large burns, consider admitting the patient to a burn center.) Discharge the patient on antibiotics—dicloxacillin (250 to 500 mg qid for 7 to 10 days), or a first-generation cephalosporin such as cephalexin (500 mg qid for 7 to 10 days). A single, parenteral dose of antibiotic followed by oral antibiotics may be used for more serious cases. The patient should return in 1 day to check for response to antibiotics. Arrangements should be made for plastic surgery wound revision in 6 to 8 months if the patient so desires.

3. Severe infection (extensive cellulitis, lymphangitis, lymphadenitis, or suppuration, often with fever or leukocytosis). The wounds should be cleaned and irrigated as with moderate infections, with a sample of pus being sent for Gram's stain and culture. All sutures should be removed. In most cases these patients should be admitted for intravenous antibiotics (cephalosporin or a penicillinase-resistant penicillin). Such infections frequently respond rapidly to antibiotics, and patients can often be discharged on oral medications within 24 hours. As in the case of moderate infections, arrangements should be made for plastic surgery wound revision in 6 to 8 months if the patient so desires.

Tissue Necrosis

Often necrosis occurs at a wound edge following suturing, especially in the case of flap lacerations. Ideally, the patient was informed at the time of suturing that the viability of the flap was in question. If, on follow-up, there are no signs of infection, the sutures should be removed and the wound allowed to heal by secondary intention. Epithelialization occurs beneath the dead tissue, and the tissue eventually peels away as an eschar. Surgical removal of the tissue is unnecessary unless the wound becomes infected. The patient should be informed about the possibility of surgical scar revision after the wound has healed.

Pain—Infection versus Neuritis

Pain in the region of a wound generally decreases as healing proceeds. Pain after 2 days thus becomes a worrisome symptom. With infections, there should be local erythema or expressible pus. Another cause of late pain is focal neuritis. Unlike infection, in which the skin near the wound is painful to light touch, with neuritis the skin in the distribution of the pain is frequently insensate. The therapy for neuritis is with a nonsteroidal anti-inflammatory drug such as ibuprofen.

Suture Removal

Suture removal should be timely enough to avoid suture marks, yet not so soon as to risk dehiscence of the wound. Table 11-2 lists times for suture removal by region. Note that early

Table 11-2 Suture Removal (Days)*

	Adults (Days)	Children (Days)
Face	4–5	3–4
Scalp	6–7	5–6
Trunk	7–10	6–8
Arm (not joints)	7–10	5–9
Leg (not joints)	8–10	6–8
Joint		
Extensor		
surface	8–14	7–12
Flexor		
surface	8–10	6–8
Dorsum of hand	7–9	5–7
Palm	7–12	7–10
Sole of foot	7–12	7–10

*Early suture removal (3–7d) should be followed by skin tape for 7–10 days. The same is also true for lacerations over the extensor surfaces of joints.

removal is recommended for the face, because this well-vascularized region heals rapidly, and hence also forms suture marks more rapidly. Children both heal faster and form suture marks faster than adults, and therefore need suture removal sooner for a given region. Following early suture removal from any area, skin tape should be applied.

Axiom: Following early suture removal, place skin tape to protect the wound.

When a patient returns for suture removal, assess the wound to be sure that it is mature enough for suture removal. If not, the patient should be instructed to return in 2 days for suture removal. When removing sutures, be certain to cut only one thread of the suture loop, and not two. Otherwise part of the suture will be retained below the skin surface (Fig. 11-2).

Scar Revision

Certain lacerations, especially those running against the normal skin tension lines, heal with unsightly scars. The scars then contract and re-

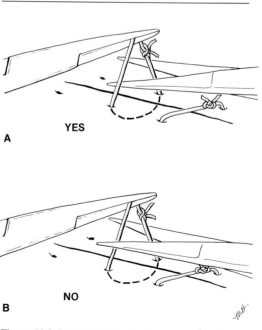

A   **YES**

B   **NO**

Figure 11-2 Suture removal. **A.** Be sure to cut only one strand of the suture loop. **B.** If both strands are mistakenly cut, suture material will be retained within the skin.

model over a period of 6 to 8 months. At the time of initial repair, patients should be informed about the possibility of scar revision after the scar has finished remodeling. Such revisions can involve excision of the scar or realignment of the scar by Z-plasty. Revisions are usually performed by the plastic surgeon.

EFFECTS OF BANDAGES AND TOPICAL AGENTS ON WOUND HEALING

Recent research has shown that bandaging materials and topical salves dramatically effect the course of healing. Lacerations and split-thickness wounds (such as blisters, abrasions, and second-degree burns) when left open to the air heal by first forming an eschar and then generating a new epidermal layer beneath the eschar. The regenerating epidermal cells must actually cleave away the overlying eschar (see Chapter 1). In wounds covered with conventional cotton gauze, the process of eschar formation proceeds unaffected. However, in wounds covered with occlusive bandages, and with certain topical salves, there is no eschar formation, epithelialization is accelerated, and the amount of scarring is often decreased.

In many of the topics discussed below, recommendations are based on data gathered from animal experimentation. Until rigorous human studies are performed, we feel that the most rational course is to extrapolate findings based on animal models to humans. Most of the products discussed are approved for human use.

Natural Healing

Uncovered Split-Thickness Injuries

Several injuries lead to a loss of some or all of the superficial epidermis, leaving intact the dermis plus epidermal appendages (hair follicles, sweat glands, sebaceous glands) that lie within the dermis. Common causes of such injuries are second-degree burns, abrasions (including graft donor sites), and blisters. Healing normally occurs by migration of epithelial cells from the

uninjured tissue at the periphery of the wound, as well as from the epidermal cells of the hair follicles, sweat, and sebaceous glands (see also Chapter 1).

After a split-thickness injury (which removes the cornified and granulosum layers, but leaves intact the dermis plus hair follicles and epidermal appendages) the superficial layers of the dermis desiccate and die. This necrotic dermal tissue becomes incorporated with dried serous fluid to form the eschar. The regenerating epithelial cells then must burrow through the junction between the healthy dermis and the necrotic cells.

Uncovered Lacerations

In sutured lacerations that are left uncovered, the superficial dermis at the wound edge desiccates and becomes necrotic, as in split-thickness injuries. Dried serous transudate, along with the desiccated dermis, forms an eschar. The epidermal cells must migrate beneath the necrotic eschar to form the new epithelial layer. After 7 days the degree of fibroplasia is significantly greater in lacerations left open to the air, compared to those covered with occlusive dressings[125] (see Fig. 11-3).

Effects of Bandaging on Wound Healing

Nonocclusive Bandages

Nonocclusive bandages, such as standard woven surgical gauze, when applied to a wound, do not effect the general pattern of healing described above for uncovered wounds.[190] There is still formation of the eschar which must be cleaved off by underlying epidermal cells.

Furthermore, surgical gauze is not a particularly effective barrier against bacterial contamination. In one study, surface bacteria were able to penetrate as many as 64 layers of gauze.[121] Occlusive bandages, however, were effective in preventing contamination.[121]

Many of the gauze bandages which for years had been considered "inert" turn out to have direct inhibitory effects on epidermal cell metabolism. The degree of tissue toxicity is gauged

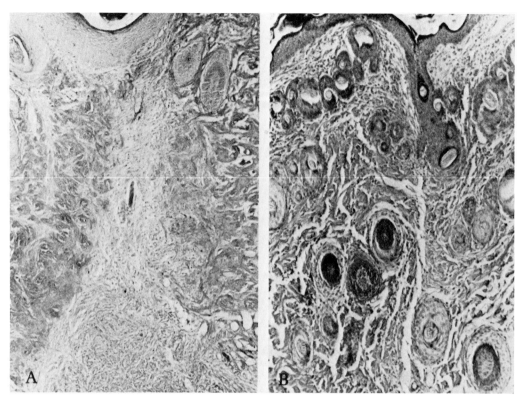

Figure 11-3 Experimental lacerations at day 7. The wound in (**A**) was left open to the air. Note the marked fibroplasia in the center of the wound. The wound in (**B**) was treated with an occlusive dressing. Note the absence of fibroplasia. *Source:* Reprinted from *The Surgical Wound* (p 195) by P Dineen and G Hildick-Smith (Eds) with permission of Lea & Febiger, © 1981.

experimentally by looking at the suppression of cell respiration engendered by various materials. Bleached cotton wool, for example, depresses cell respiration by 15 percent, standard hospital-grade cotton wool by to 20 percent, and standard woven surgical gauze caused a 20 percent reduction.

The primary drawback of using gauze and other nonocclusive bandages as direct wound coverings is the problem of adherence to the wound. As the serous material dries, the gauze becomes incorporated into the crust. Hence, removal of the dressing becomes a tedious and painful process. Frequently, as the bandage is removed, the adhering eschar comes off as well, and with it the newly formed epithelial layer as well.[190] Another problem with gauze is that bits of lint flake off and can actually cause a foreign body reaction in the healing tissue.[121] Bandages made of nonadherent material but with multiple

fenestrations also adhere, because serous material dries and crusts at the fenestrations. In summary, nonocclusive dressings tend to adhere to the wound surface, and may actually have direct, inhibitory effects on wound healing.

Occlusive (Nonadherent) Bandages

In experimental animal abrasions treated with occlusive dressings, such as polyurethane film, heal more rapidly than in uncovered control wounds. In one study, by the third day almost all wounds in the occlusive dressing group had regenerated a new epidermal layer, compared to none in the control group (see Table 11-3).[47]

There is also new evidence that occlusive bandages may speed healing in lacerations.[125] However, there is conflicting data on the effect of occlusive dressings on the tensile strength of healing lacerations.[14]

Table 11-3 Comparison of Occlusive Polyethylene Film Bandage to Unbandaged Controls in the Healing of Experimental Abrasions

Time postwound (days)	2	3	4	5	6	7
Control (%)	0[a]	0	33	94	100	100
Polyethylene (%)	0	86	90	100	100	100

Source: Adapted from *The Surgical Wound* by P Dineen and G Hildick-Smith (Eds) with permission of Lea & Febiger, © 1981.

[a]The numbers refer to the percentage of wounds in each group that had a complete epithelial layer at the time indicated.

Some authors report increased bacteria counts under occlusive dressings, while others found decreased counts.[121,158] Investigators who note decreased bacterial counts in experimental wounds treated with occlusion reason that there is less necrotic skin, and that white blood cells are able to move more easily to phagocytose invading organisms.[121] In a study of human lacerations, there was no significant difference in the wound infection rate between those treated with occlusive as opposed to aerated dressings.[186] In the same study, patients treated with occlusive dressings reported significantly less wound discomfort than those bandaged with nonocclusive dressings.[186]

There are many occlusive dressings now on the market. The authors prefer conventional polyurethane film (OpSite, Tegaderm, Biocclusive) and occlusive foams (Primaderm, Duoderm) which are easy to use and relatively inexpensive. Some of the biologic dressings are prohibitively expensive, and have not been shown to be superior to conventional polyurethane film.

Summary

Occlusive bandages have several advantages over nonocclusive bandages. Occlusive bandages do not adhere to the wound, hence dressing changes are easier. In both split-thickness injuries and in sutured lacerations, occlusive dressings significantly speed epithelialization, while at the same time decreasing desiccation and necrosis of the dermis. The end result is a wound that heals faster and with less scar tissue. The long-term effects of occlusive bandages on wound tensile strength remains to be determined.

Effects of Topical Medications on Wound Healing

For many years humans have sought a topical balm that would accelerate wound healing:

> A Samaritan, as he journeyed . . . went to him and bound up his wounds, pouring on oil. (*Luke* 10:33)

As noted above, many bandaging materials have favorable effects on wound healing. Topical creams and salves have also been found to alter the course of wound healing. Several agents, such as Silvadene and Neosporin ointment, speed epithelialization. Other agents, such as standard USP petrolatum, may actually retard healing. In many cases the effects on healing are produced by the vehicle of the ointment or cream, and not by the "active" ingredients.

Inert Creams, Lotions, and Salves

Based on the improved wound healing afforded by occlusive bandages, one would expect that USP petrolatum would also improve healing. Amazingly, standard petrolatum actually retards healing in experimental animals. In split-thickness lesions in animals, epithelialization took significantly longer in wounds treated with USP petrolatum as opposed to control subjects as shown in Table 11-4. Note that on day 5, whereas more than two-thirds of control subjects' wounds had a full epithelial layer, in

Table 11-4 Comparison of USP Petrolatum to Control Subjects in the Healing of Experimental Abrasions

Time postwound (days)	2	3	4	5	6	7
Control (%)	0[a]	6	20	70	100	100
USP petrolatum (%)	0	8	10	30	83	88

Source: Adapted from *The Surgical Wound* by P Dineen and G Hildick-Smith (Eds) with permission of Lea & Febiger, © 1981.

[a]The numbers refer to the percentage of wounds in each group that had a complete epidermal layer at the time indicated.

the USP petrolatum group fewer than one-third had a complete layer.

Although standard petrolatum retards healing, in similar experiments, low-melting-point petrolatum, which is the vehicle for Neosporin ointment, does not retard healing.[47] Water-miscible creams (such as the "inert" vehicle of Silvadene) actually speed healing by as much as 25 percent.[47]

Topical Antibacterial Agents

Several antibacterial products are available for application to wounds. These agents have varying effects upon healing. Neosporin ointment is a combination of neomycin, polymyxin, and bacitracin, in a low melting-point petrolatum base. In animals, Neosporin significantly increases the rate of epithelialization of experimental split-thickness wounds, by up to 25 percent.[47] Silvadene cream speeds experimental healing by 28 percent over control animals but this is not significantly better than the improvement gained by the plain cream vehicle without the active ingredient silver sulfadiazine.[47] Povidone-iodine ointment neither speeds nor retards healing.[47] Furacin, another topical antimicrobial agent, retards healing by as much as 30 percent.[47] Table 11-5 compares the number of days until 50 percent of experimental wounds are healed (the HT_{50}) for antibiotic topical agent, the plain vehicle, and untreated control subjects.[47]

Summary

Various topical aftercare agents have different effects on experimental wound healing. Both Silvadene and Neosporin speed healing. Furacin

retards healing, and Pharmadine ointment appears to have no effect. Adequate human experimentation remains to be done.

The authors recommend the use of Neosporin ointment, which is both inexpensive and easy to apply. We have also had good outcomes using bacitracin ointment (not tested in animal studies). Bacitracin ointment may have less potential for allergic reactions than Neosporin.[145]

BANDAGING TECHNIQUE[136,180]

This section deals with basic bandaging techniques, first according to the configuration of the

Table 11-5 Effects of Antimicrobial Agents and Their "Inert" Vehicles on Wound Healing

Agent	HT_{50} (days)	Healing Rate Relative to Control Subjects
Neosporin	3.6	+ 25
Vehicle	4.6	+ 4
Control	4.8	0
Pharmadine	4.6	0
Control	4.6	0
Furacin	6.0	− 30
Vehicle	4.8	− 4
Control	4.8	0
Silvadene	3.1	+ 28
Vehicle	3.4	+ 21
Control	4.3	0

Source: Adapted from *The Surgical Wound* by P Dineen and G Hildick-Smith (Eds) with permission of Lea & Febiger, © 1981.

dressing and then according to the region to be wrapped. The basic configurations are the circular wrap, the simple spiral, the reversed spiral, and the figure-eight wrap. The section on regional bandaging displays and discusses dressings for various areas of the body, such as head and neck, trunk, and extremities. The dressings can be used for bandaging lacerations, abrasions, and burns alike.

Basic Bandaging

Primary Dressing

In all the bandages described below, first a primary dressing is placed directly over the wound. As noted in Effects of Bandages and Topical Agents on Wound Healing, above, the primary dressing should be occlusive in nature. In most cases the primary dressing consists of a vapor-permeable occlusive dressing such as polyurethane film, with an overlying absorbent pad, or an antimicrobial salve. Such a dressing allows for drainage of wound exudate, while at the same time suppressing formation of the eschar (Fig. 11-4).

In areas of the body where a bandage would tend to shift positions easily, such as the upper lip, a topical antiseptic salve alone, such as Neosporin or bacitracin, can be spread over the wound, as shown in Figure 11-5. The patient should be instructed to reapply the salve approximately every 4 hours while awake.

Secondary Dressing

General. After the primary bandage has been placed, the secondary bandage is wrapped over it to keep it in place. The most commonly used materials are rolls of plain cotton gauze of various widths. Innumerable other suitable bandaging materials are available, including thickly fluffed rolled gauze (Kerlex), elastic bandages (Ace wraps), and adherent elastic bandages (Elastoplast).

After the secondary bandage is complete, either plastic or cloth tape can be used to keep it in place.

Simple Gauze Bandage. For small wounds a simple 2-inch or 4-inch square of gauze can be placed over the primary dressing (either topical salve or occlusive dressing) and taped into position. The gauze can be filled (ideal for wounds that ooze such as abrasions) or unfilled.

The gauze can be laid down without folding to cover a square lesion. Alternately, the gauze can be folded in half to create a rectangular bandage, as shown in Figure 11-6.

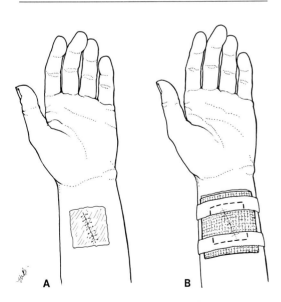

Figure 11-4 Method of applying occlusive dressing. Applying the dressing against the skin, and holding it in place with conventional gauze allows secretions to escape around the edges of the dressing and not pool around the wound.

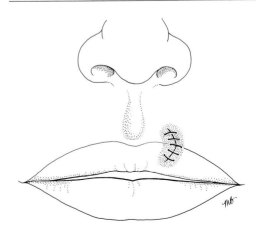

Figure 11-5 A topical antimicrobial salve can be used to cover regions such as the lip where conventional bandaging is not practical.

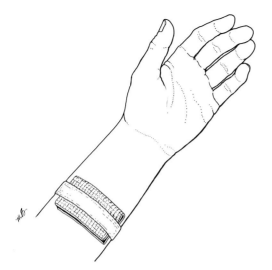

Figure 11-6 Simple gauze bandage. See text for discussion.

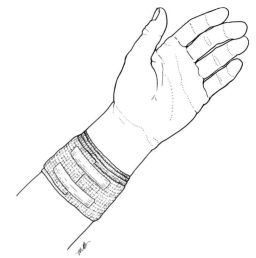

Figure 11-7 The circular bandage.

The Circular Bandage. The circular bandage, one of the most commonly used bandages, is also one of the easiest to make. The bandage is simply wrapped around the injured region a total of two to three layers and then taped in place, as shown in Figure 11-7. Cylindrical regions of the body are most amenable to this type of wrap.

The Simple Spiral Bandage. The simple spiral wrap can be used for wrapping either cylindrical and conical regions of the body. First, the bandage is secured by making a two-layer circular wrap at the base of the region to be dressed. Then the wrap is rolled up or down to cover the injured area. The wrap should be made to overlap itself by 40 to 50 percent with each turn of the spiral, as shown in Figure 11-8. The bandage is completed by making a single layer circular wrap and taping it in place.

The simple spiral bandage is best suited for cylindrical regions of the body. For conical regions, such as the thigh, the dressing has a tendency to slip down toward the apex of the cone. Using an elastic bandage decreases the chances of having the bandage slip out of place.

Reversed Spiral Bandage. The reversed spiral bandage is suited for conical regions of the body such as the forearm and thigh. The reversed spiral stays in position better than the simple spiral dressing but is also harder to wrap. First

wrap twice circumferentially, then angle either up or down, go halfway around from back to front, then anchor the bandage with a thumb, fold back the bandage over the thumb, and repeat (Fig. 11-9).

Taping Technique

Avoid tight, constricting circular bands of tape around extremities. In the event of swelling, excess tape increases distal edema and may even diminish arterial flow. Either use ¾ circles or the spiral technique.

Adhesive tape rips easily if first distracted and then torn, as illustrated in Figure 11-10.

Pressure Dressings

A small amount of pressure over the wounded area serves to decrease local edema as well as to enhance hemostasis. Hence pressure is especially advantageous in deep wounds to help obliterate dead space. Adequate pressure can be obtained by placing three gauze pads over the primary dressing, and wrapping the final layer with an elastic bandage.

Splints

Lacerations over joints heal better if splinted for 5 days. Conventional plaster gauze can be employed, using 8 to 10 layers for the upper

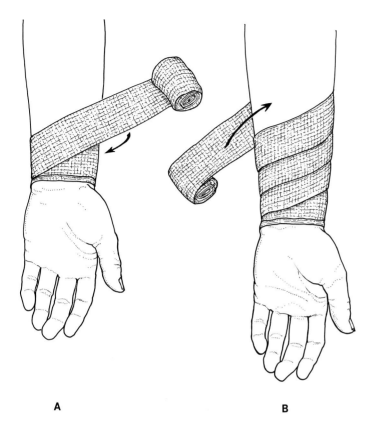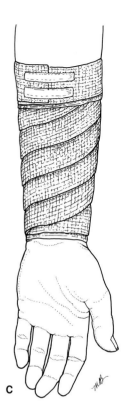

A   **B**   **C**

Figure 11-8 The spiral bandage. See text for discussion.

extremity and 10 to 12 layers for the lower extremity.

Atlas of Regional Bandaging

This section displays and discusses dressings for various regions of the body. The dressings can be used for bandaging lacerations, abrasions, and burns alike.

Scalp

For wounds on the top (or vertex) of the skull, a topical antibacterial ointment alone is usually sufficient (see above).

For extensive vertex laceration, a complete head dressing can be applied. The bandage is initially secured with a circular wrap around the skull, then the bandage is run forward and backward over the vertex until the wound is ade-

quately covered. Finally, another circular wrap is applied and taped into position at the brow[180] (Fig. 11-11). The dressing should be snug but not so tight as to cause discomfort. The ears must be padded or excluded to prevent discomfort or necrosis.

Wounds along the periphery of the scalp can be covered with a simple circular wrap. Small scalp lacerations can be dressed with an antibiotic ointment alone.

Forehead

Large forehead wounds, especially deep lacerations, should be wrapped with a simple circular bandage extending all the way around the head. The pressure afforded by the circular wrap keeps the dead space closed and reduces wound edema.

Smaller wounds can be treated with a simple gauze bandage.

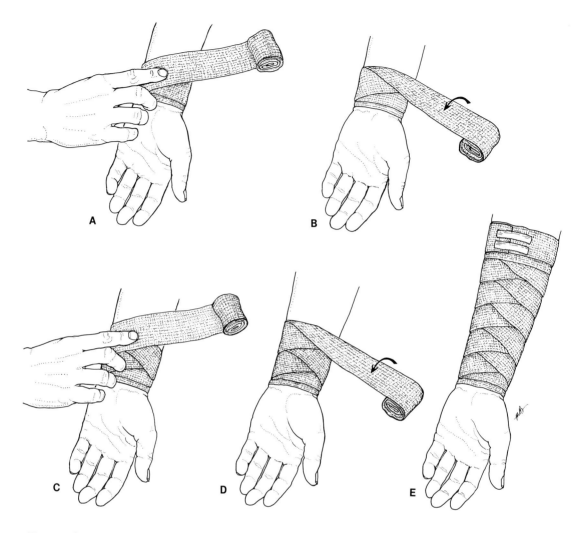

Figure 11-9 The reversed spiral bandage. See text for discussion.

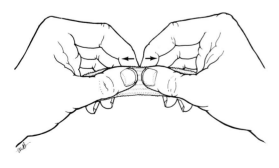

Figure 11-10 Distracting cloth tape prior to tearing makes tearing more easy.

Ear

For major ear injuries, especially those involving the cartilage, an ear splint should be formed, as illustrated in Figure 11-12. First apply an antibiotic ointment over the entire extent of the laceration. Next form a cast of the anterior part of the ear using moistened cotton wool. Then bolster the posterior aspect of the ear using either two or three fluffs of plain gauze or moistened cotton wool. Finally, wrap the entire bandage into place using a circular bandage around the head. This pressure dressing maintains the architecture of the ear during healing,

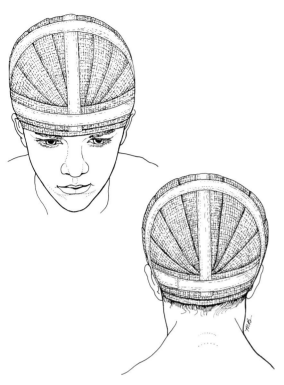

and helps guard against the formation of hematomas (see also Chapter 8).

Small wounds of the ear are most easily managed with frequent reapplications of antibiotic ointment.

Eyebrow

Bandaging in the eyebrow region is frequently neglected because such bandages are unsightly. However, especially with deep lacerations, the physician should advise the patient that it is better to endure a few days with a clumsy dressing than many years with an unnecessarily thickened scar.

For deep lacerations, the eyebrow should be dressed first with antibiotic ointment, since a simple occlusive bandage does not adequately guard against the formation of an eschar beneath the hairs. Next, overlay a folded gauze square. The entire bandage is then secured with a simple circular wrap around the head, as shown in Figure 11-13.

For small lacerations or abrasions, frequent applications of antibiotic ointment can be used in lieu of the large dressing.

Figure 11-11 Scalp bandage for extensive scalp lacerations. The posterior portion of the wrap should reach below the occipital prominence to help secure the dressing into place. When possible, leave openings for the ears.

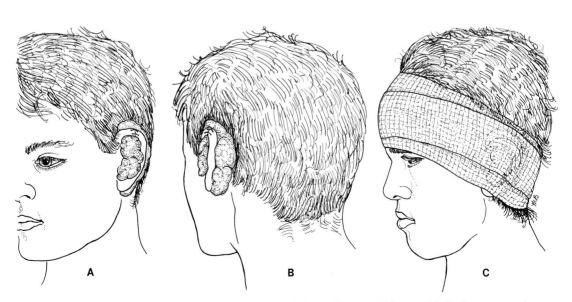

Figure 11-12 The ear splint. Moistened cotton wool is used to pack the anterior aspect of the ear and fluffs of gauze are used to bolster the posterior aspect. The splint is kept in position with a circular bandage around the head.

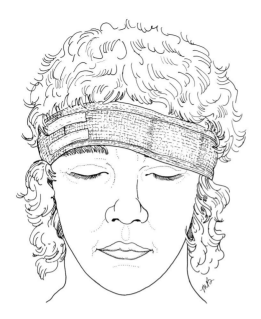

Figure 11-13 Eyebrow bandage. See text for discussion.

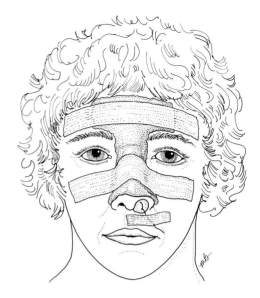

Figure 11-14 Special dressing for extensive nasal lacerations that involve cartilage. The packing in each nostril consists of Xeroform gauze wrapped around cotton balls. A length of suture is tied around each packing to aid in removal. The outer splint is made of plaster of paris (six layers of standard casting plaster gauze).

Nose

Most dressings for the nose can consist of a simple bandage which arcs over the injured area and which is then affixed with tape to the cheeks on both sides.

A special dressing, which has both nasal packs and a splint, is necessary for extensive nasal lacerations that involve the cartilage (Fig. 11-14). In these cases a pack consisting of a small oval sphere constructed by wrapping Xeroform gauze over a small cotton ball should be inserted into the nares to maintain the shape of the nose during healing. A length of suture material is tied around the pack and taped to the upper lip, to aid in subsequent removal of the pack. The outer portion of the laceration is covered with either an occlusive bandage such as polyurethane film or an antibiotic ointment. A piece of gauze is placed over the primary dressing, and the entire nose is splinted with a small cast consisting of six layers of regular casting material. Prefabricated nasal splints are available as well.

Cheek

Cheek injuries can be dressed with a simple gauze bandage. If pressure is required, place a

strip of Elastoplast over a folded piece of gauze, as illustrated in Figure 11-15.

Lip

Lip injuries are not amenable to standard bandages. However, the injured region can be protected against desiccation and infection by the frequent application of a topical ointment such as bacitracin or Neomycin. Patients should be educated to apply the ointment every 2 to 3 hours while awake.

Chin

The chin can be bandaged with a simple rectangular gauze dressing. As described for the cheek, Elastoplast can be used to make a pressure dressing.

Neck

Most neck injuries can be covered with a simple gauze bandage. One should avoid circumferential gauze or tape, because of the pos-

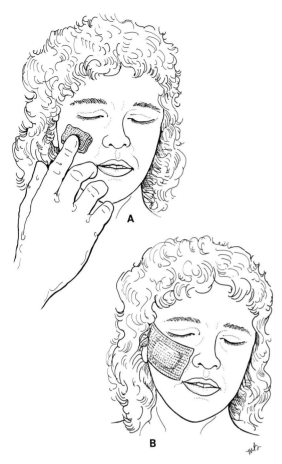

Figure 11-15 A. A piece of folded gauze is placed over the primary dressing. **B.** Next, elastoplast is applied.

sibility of compression on vessels and airway if swelling occurs.

Upper Extremity

Upper Arm or Forearm. The upper arm or forearm can be bandaged with a simple ascending spiral, a reversed spiral, or circular wrap.

Elbow. The bandaging technique for the elbow varies according to whether the elbow is to be splinted straight or flexed (remember, lacerations at joints should be splinted for the first 5 days).

To dress the elbow when the arm is to be held straight, use a circular wrap. When the arm is flexed to 90 degrees, however, the best bandage is a figure-eight (Fig. 11-16). Begin at the fore-

arm portion, with a simple circular wrap to secure the bandage. Next cover the olecranon, and wrap back in a figure-eight fashion to the forearm. A similar maneuver is then used to bandage the area below and above the olecranon proper. The dressing is secured with a circular wrap on the upper arm.

Antecubital Fossa. The antecubital fossa can be wrapped with a figure-eight bandage, as shown in Figure 11-17.

Wrist. Wrist injuries can be covered with a simple circular gauze wrap.

Dorsal Hand. The dorsum of the hand can be dressed with either a simple gauze bandage for small injuries, or a figure-eight bandage for larger injuries.

For the figure-eight dressing, begin with a circular wrap at the wrist. Then go up and around the hand and back around the wrist two or three times until the desired area is adequately covered, as shown in Figure 11-18.

Palm. Simple injuries of the palm can be covered the same as dorsal hand injuries described above.

If more protection is needed, make a bulky hand dressing by fluffing several pieces of gauze between the fingers and then over the palm. Then use plain circular gauze or an elastic bandage to secure the fluffs into position as shown in Figure 11-19.

Finger. Small wounds of the fingers can be covered with either a plain Band-Aid or a simple gauze dressing. Larger injuries can be dressed with either tube gauze or a figure-eight wrap between the finger and the wrist.

When using tube gauze, remember that tube gauze should *never* be twisted at the base of the finger, but only at the finger tip. Twisting at the base of a finger can cause disastrous strangulation of the blood supply with possible loss of the digit.

The figure-eight bandage begins with a circular wrap of the wrist, starting on the ulnar aspect and then wrapping along the volar aspect to the radius, and around a full circle, ending at the radial aspect (Fig. 11-20). Then track dorsally across the back of the hand, aiming for the

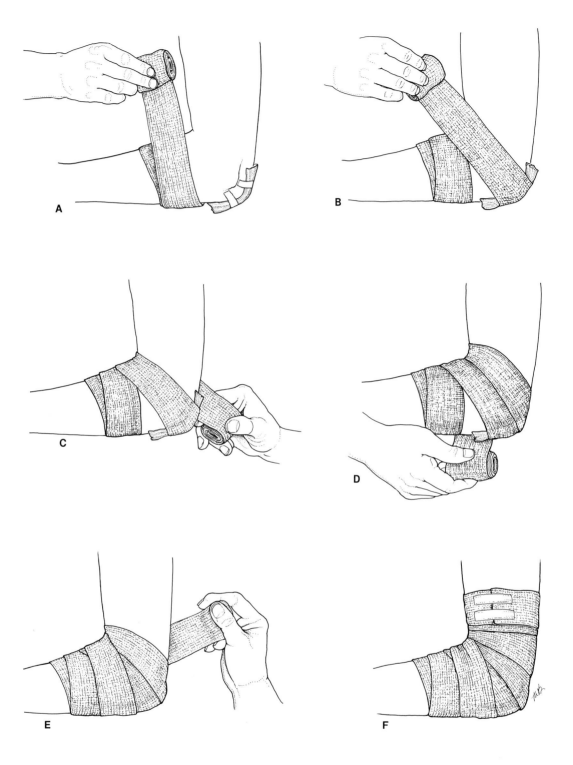

Figure 11-16 Figure-eight elbow wrap. Start with a circular wrap on the proximal forearm (**A**). Then wrap around the olecranon (**B**) and back to the forearm (**C**). Make additional wraps both below (C) and above the olecranon. And finally end with a two-layer circular wrap on the upper arm (**D**).

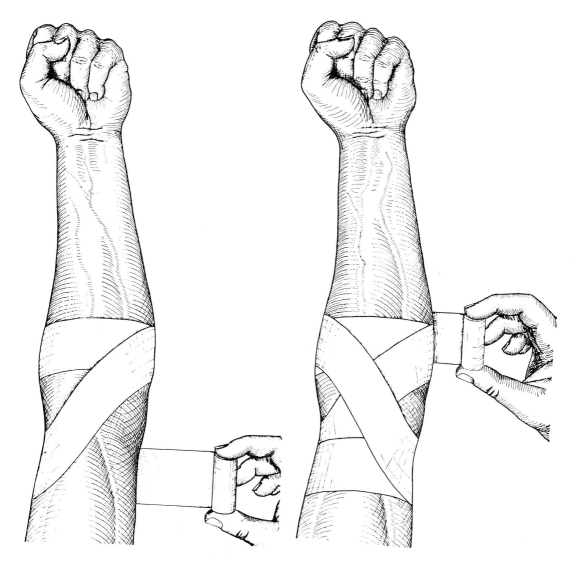

Figure 11-17 Figure-eight wrap of the antecubital fossa. *Source:* Reprinted from *A Manual of Bandaging, Strapping and Splinting,* ed 3 (pp 58–59) by A Thorndike with permission of Lea & Febiger, © 1959.

afflicted digit. Use an ascending and then a descending spiral to wrap the finger, and finish by angling across the dorsum of hand to the ulna and secure with a circular wrist wrap.[136]

A similar technique can be used to wrap the thumb.

Lower Extremity

Thigh. The thigh is conical in shape and can be wrapped with either a simple gauze square for small injuries or a spiral wrap for larger dressings.

Knee. The knee is usually wrapped with the leg straight so that the patient can walk. A simple circular or ascending spiral bandage will suffice.

Lower Leg. The lower leg, like the thigh, is conical in shape and can be wrapped with either a simple gauze square for small injuries or a spiral wrap for larger dressings.

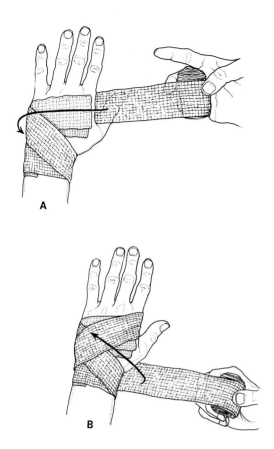

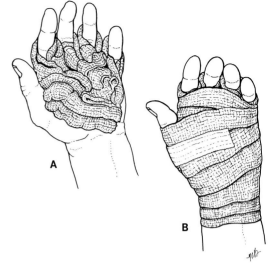

Figure 11-19 Bulky hand dressing for palm injuries. **A.** First fluffs of plain gauze are placed between the fingers. **B.** Gauze is then used to hold the dressing in place. This dressing can also be used for injuries to the dorsal hand and proximal phalanges.

Ankle or Heel. Injuries of the ankle or the heel are most easily wrapped with a modified figure-eight technique, illustrated in Figure 11-21. The wrap is initially secured with a circular wrap around the lower leg at the level of the malleoli. Then the wrap is circled first around the heel, and then back and forth in a figure-eight fashion around the ankle and foot.

Foot. Wounds of both the dorsum and the sole of the foot can be covered using a simple circular gauze wrap. The wrap should not be too bulky because bulky wraps are uncomfortable to walk on.

Toes. The toes can be wrapped with either a simple Band-Aid or gauze square, or with either tube gauze or a spiral wrap as described above for finger dressings. The injured toe can be immobilized by taping it to an adjacent toe. Cotton should be placed between the two toes to avoid maceration.

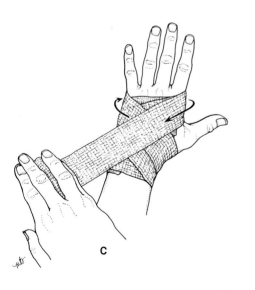

Figure 11-18 Dorsal hand wrap. See text for discussion.

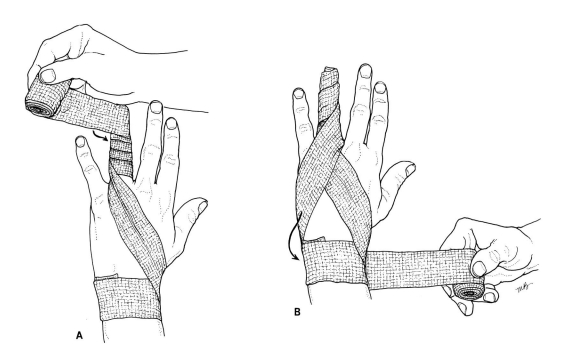

Figure 11-20 Finger bandage. **A.** Begin with a circular wrap around the wrist. **B.** Then cross the dorsal hand and ascend the finger with a spiral wrap. **C.** Next spiral down the finger and angle back over the hand to end with a circular wrap at the wrist.

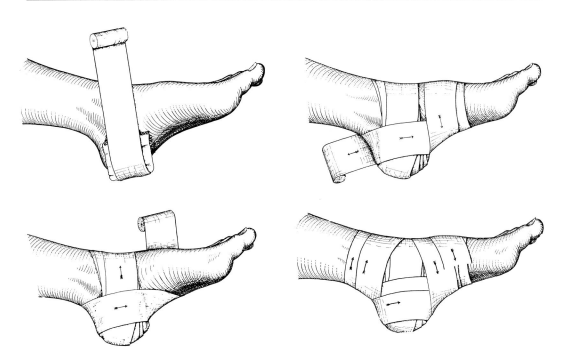

Figure 11-21 Modified figure-eight wrap for ankle and heel injuries. See text for discussion. *Source:* Reprinted from *A Manual of Bandaging, Strapping and Splinting*, ed 3 (pp 64–65) by A Thorndike with permission of Lea & Febiger, © 1959.

Bibliography

1. Adams IW: A comparative trial of polyglycolic acid and silk as suture materials for accidental wounds. *Lancet* 1977;1216.

2. Aghababian RV, Conte JE: Mammalian bite wounds. *Ann Emerg Med* 1980;9:79.

3. Alexander JW, Kaplan JZ, Altemeier WA: Role of suture materials in the development of wound infection. *Ann Surg* 1967;165:192.

4. Allen MJ: Conservative management of finger tip injuries in adults. *Hand* 1980;12:257.

5. Anderson MA, Newmeyer WL, Kilgore ES Jr: Diagnosis and treatment of retained foreign bodies in the hand. *Am J Surg* 1982;144:63.

6. Ariyan S: A simple stereotactic method to isolate and remove foreign bodies. *Arch Surg* 1977;112:857.

7. Ashbell TS, Kleinert HE, Putcha SM, et al.: The deformed finger nail, a frequent result of failure to repair nail bed injuries. *J Trauma* 1967;7:177.

8. Bauer AR, Yutani D: Computed Tomographic localization of wooden foreign bodies in children's extremities. *Arch Surg* 1983;118:1084.

9. Berkelman RL, Holland BW, Anderson RL: Increased bactericidal activity of dilute preparations of povidone-iodine solutions. *Clin Micro* 1982;15:635.

10. Borges AF, Alexander FE, Black LI: Z-plasty treatment of unesthetic scars. *Eye Ear Nose Throat Monthly* 1965;44:39.

11. Borges AF, Alexander JE: Relaxed skin tension lines. Z-plasties on scars, and fusiform excision of lesions. *Br J Plastic Surg* 1962;15:242.

12. Bormley DE: Use of Burow's wedge principle for repair of wounds in or near the eyebrow. *J Am Acad Dermatol* 1985;12:344.

13. Boss WK, Brand DA, Acampora D, et al.: Effectiveness of prophylactic antibiotics in the outpatient treatment of burns. *J Trauma* 1985;25:224.

14. Bothwell JW, Rovee DT: The effects of dressings on the repair of cutaneous wounds in humans. In Harkiss KJ (ed): *Surgical Dressings and Wound Healing*. London: Bradford University Press, 1971.

15. Brand RA, Black H: Pseudomonas osteomyelitis following puncture wounds in children. *J Bone Joint Surg* 1974;56-A:1637.

16. Branemark PI, Ekholm R, Albrektsson B, et al.: Tissue injury caused by wound disinfectants. *J Bone Joint Surg* 1967;49-A:48.

17. Brody GS, Cloutier AM, Woolhouse FG: The finger tip injury—an assessment of management. *Plast Reconstruct Surg* 1960;26:81.

18. Brown CG, Ashton JJ: Dog bites, the controversy continues. *Am J Emerg Med* 1985;3:83.

19. Brown LL, Shelton HT, Bornside GH, et al.: Evaluation of wound irrigation by pulsatile jet and conventional methods. *Ann Surg* 1978;187:170.

20. Bryant CA, Rodeheaver GT, Reem EM, et al.: Search for a nontoxic surgical scrub solution for periorbital lacerations. *Ann Emerg Med* 1984;13:317.

21. Buck JK, Spotte S, Gadbaw JJ: Bacteriology of the teeth from a great white shark: Potential medical implications for shark bite victims. *J Clin Microbiol* 1984;20:849.

22. Burdge DR, Scheifele D, Speert DP: Serious *Pasteurella multocida* infections from lion and tiger bites. *JAMA* 1985;253:3296.

23. Caldwell DR, Kastl PR, Cook J, et al.: Povidone-Iodine: Its efficacy as a preoperative conjunctival and periocular preparation. *Ann Ophthalmol* 1984;16:579.

24. Callaham M: Dog bite wounds. *JAMA* 1980; 244:2327.

25. Callaham M: Prophylactic antibiotics in common dog bite wounds: A controlled study. *Ann Emerg Med* 1980; 9:410.

26. Callaham ML: Treatment of common dog bites: Infection risk factors. *J Am Coll Emerg Phys* 1978;7:83.

27. Carithers HA: Diagnosis of cat-scratch disease. *Pediatrics* 1985;76:325.

28. Chun YT, Berkelhamer JE, Herold TE: Dog bites in children less than 4 years old. *Pediatrics* 1982;69:119.

29. Chusid MJ, Jacobs WM, Sty JR: Pseudomonas arthritis following puncture wounds of the foot. *J Pediatr* 1979;94:429.

30. Clark RAF: Cutaneous tissue repair: Basic biologic considerations. I. *Am Acad Dermatol* 1985;13:701.

31. Cohen AM: Core clinical clerkship EW procedures—Massachusetts General Hospital, 1978. (In-hospital publication.)

32. Cohen BE, Cronin ED: An innervated cross-finger flap for fingertip reconstruction. *Plast Reconstruct Surg* 1983;72:688.

33. Cracciolo A: Wooden foreign bodies in the foot. *Am J Surg* 1980;140:586.

34. Crikelair GF: Skin suture marks. *Am J Surg* 1958; 96:631.

35. Crissman RK: Punctures through sneakers (letter). *Hosp Pract* 1983;18:21.

36. Crosby SA, Powell DA: The potential value of the sedimentation rate in monitoring treatment outcome in puncture wound-related pseudomonas osteomyelitis. *Clin Orthop Rel Res* 1984;188:168.

37. Curtin JW: Basic plastic surgical techniques in repair of facial lacerations. *Surg Clin North Am* 1973;53:33.

38. Custer J, Edlich RF, Prusak M, et al.: Studies in the management of the contaminated wound V. An assessment of the effectiveness of Phisohex and Betadine surgical scrub solutions. *Am J Surg* 1971;121:572.

39. Das De S, McAllister TA: Pseudomonas osteomyelitis following puncture wounds of the foot in children. *Injury* 1981;12:334.

40. De Jong TE, Vierhout RJ, van Vroonhoven TJ: Povidone-iodine irrigation of the subcutaneous tissue to prevent surgical wound infections. *Surg Gynecol Obstet* 1982; 155:221.

41. Denver General Hospital, Department of Emergency Medicine: Lacerations, Assessment and Repair. January 17, 1986. (In-house publication)

42. Dineen P, Hildick-Smith G: The surgical wound. Philadelphia: Lea & Febiger, 1981.

43. Douglas BS: Conservative management of guillotine amputation of the finger in children. *Aust Pediatr J* 1972;8:86.

44. DuMortier JJ: Resistance of healing wounds to infection. *Surg Gyn Obstet* 1933;56:762.

45. Dushoff IM: About face. *Emerg Med* 1974;25.

46. Dushoff IM: ''A stitch in time.'' *Emerg Med* 1983;1.

47. Eaglstein WH, Mertz PM: Effects of topical medicaments on the rate of repair of superficial wounds. In Dineen P, Hildick-Smith G (eds): *The Surgical Wound.* Philadelphia: Lea & Febiger, 1981, pp 150–170.

48. Earley MJ, Bardsley AF: Human bites: A review. *Br J Plast Surg* 1985;37:458.

49. Edlich RF, Madden JE, Prusak M, et al.: Studies in the management of the contaminated wound: VI. The therapeutic value of gentle scrubbing in prolonging the limited period of effectiveness of antibiotics in contaminated wounds. *Am J Surg* 1971;121:668.

50. Edlich RF, Panek PH, Rodeheaver GT, et al.: Physical and chemical configuration of sutures in the development of surgical infection. *Ann Surg* 1972;177:679.

51. Edlich RF, Rodeheaver GT, Horowitz JH, et al.: Emergency department management of puncture wounds and needlestick exposures. *Emerg Med Clin North Am* 1986;4:581.

52. Edlich RF, Rodeheaver GT, Thacker JG, et al.: Fundamentals of wound management in surgery—technical factors in wound management. South Plainfield, NJ: Chirugecom;1977.

53. Edlich RF, Smith QT, Edgerton MT: Resistance of the surgical wound to antimicrobial prophylaxis and its mechanisms of development. *Am J Surg* November 1973;126:583.

54. Edlich RF, Tsung M, Rogers W, et al.; Studies in management of the contaminated wound. 1. Technique of closure. *J Surg Res* 1968;8:585.

55. Elek SD, Conen PE: The virulence of *Staphylococcos pyogenes* for man. Study of the problems of wound infection. *Br J Exp Pathol* 1957;38:573.

56. Elenbaas RM, McNabney WK, Robinson WA: Evaluation of prophylactic oxacillin in cat bite wounds. *Ann Emerg Med* 1984;13:155.

57. Elenbaas RM, McNabney WK, Robinson WA: Prophylactic oxacillin in dog bite wounds. *Ann Emerg Med* 1982;11:248.

58. Elliot DL, Tolle SW, Goldberg L, et al.: Pet-associated illness. *N Engl J Med* 1985;313:985.

59. Elliot SF, Aronoff SC: Clinical presentation and management of Pseudomonas osteomyelitis. *Clin Pediatr* 1985;24:566.

60. Epstein E: The buried horizontal mattress suture. *Cutis* 1979;24:104.

61. Ermerson EB: Fishhooks. *NY St J Med* 1966;2414.

62. Faddis D, Daniel D, Boyer J: Tissue toxicity of antiseptic solutions: A study of rabbit articular and periarticular tissues. *J Trauma* 1977;17:895.

63. Farrell RG, Disher WA, Nesland RS, et al.: Conservative management of fingertip amputations. *JACEP* 1977; 6:243.

64. Farrior RT, Jarchow RC, Rojas B: Primary and late plastic repair of soft tissue injuries. *Otolaryngol Clin North Am* 1983;16:697.

65. Fasting OJ, Bjerkreim I: Polyglycolic acid, Dexon subcuticular suture in paediatric orthopaedic surgery. *Acta Chir Scand* 1981;147:509–511.

66. Faust RA, Roy WA, Ewin DM, et al.: Management and tetanus prophylaxis in the treatment of puncture wounds. *Am Surg* 1972;38:198.

67. Fisher MC, Goldsmith JF, Gilligan PH: Sneakers as a source of *Pseudomonas aeruginosa* in children with osteomyelitis following puncture wounds. *J Pediatr* 1985; 106:607.

68. Fitzgerald RH, Cowan JDE: Puncture wounds of the foot. *Orthop Clin North Am* 1975;6:965.

69. Fox JW, Golden GT, Rodeheaver G, et al.: Non-operative Management of Fingertip pulp amputation by occlusive dressings. *Am J Surg* 1977;133:255.

70. Francis DP, Holmes MA, Brandon G: *Pasteurella multocida* infections after domestic animal bites and scratches. *JAMA* 1975;233:42.

71. Gahhos F, Arons M: Soft-tissue foreign body removal: Management and presentation of a new technique. *J Trauma* 1984;24:340.

72. Geogiade NG, Harris WA: Open and closed treatment of burns with povidone-iodine. *Plast Reconstruct Surg* 1973;52:640.

73. Geronemus RG, Mertz PM, Eaglestein WH: Wound healing: The effects of topical antimicrobial agents. *Arch Dermatol* 1979;115:1311.

74. Giffin GS: The wrestler's ear (acute auricular hematoma). *Arch Otolaryngol* 1985;111:161.

75. Gilmore GJ, Sanderson PJ: Prophylactic interparietal povidone-iodine in abdominal surgery. *Br J Surg* 1975;62:792.

76. Gilmore OJ, Reid C, Strokon A: A study of the effect of povidone-iodine on wound healing. *Postgrad Med J* 1977;53:122.

77. Glotzer DJ, Goodman WS, Lippman HG, et al.: Topical antibiotic prophylaxis in contaminated wounds. *Arch Surg* 1970;100:589.

78. Gnann JW, Bressler GS, Bodet CA, et al.: Human blastomycosis after a dog bite. *Ann Intern Med* 1983;98:48.

79. Goldberg HM, Rosenthal SA, Nemetz JC: Effect of washing closed head and neck wounds on wound healing and infection. *Am J Surg* 1981;141:358.

80. Goldstein EJC, Citron DM, Finegold SM: Dog bite wounds and infection: A prospective clinical study. *Ann Emerg Med* 1980;9:508.

81. Grabb WC, Smith JW: *Plastic Surgery*, ed 3. Boston: Little, Brown, 1979.

82. Graham BS, Gregory DW: *Pseudomonas aeruginosa* causing osteomyelitis after puncture wounds of the foot. *South Med J* 1984;177:1228.

83. Green NE, Bruno J: Pseudomonas infections of the foot after puncture wounds. *South Med J* 1980;73:146.

84. Green NE: Pseudomonas infections of the foot following puncture wounds. *Instr Course Lect* 1983;32:43.

85. Gross A, Cutright DE, Surindar BG, et al.: Effectiveness of pulsating water jet lavage in treatment of contaminated crushed wounds. *Am J Surg* 1972;124:373.

86. Grossman JA: *Minor Injuries and Disorders: Surgical and Medical Care*. Philadelphia: JB Lippincott, 1984.

87. Grossman JAI, Adams JP, Kunec J: Prophylactic antibiotics in simple hand lacerations. *JAMA* 1981; 245:1055.

88. Hagler DJ: Pseudomonas osteomyelitis: Puncture wounds of the feet (LTR). *Pediatr* 1971;48:678.

89. Halasz NA: Wound infection and topical antibiotics. *Arch Surg* 1977;112:1240.

90. Hamer ML, Robson MC, Krizek TJ, et al.: Quantitative bacterial analysis of comparative wound irrigation. *Ann Surg* 1975;181:819.

91. Harkiss KH (ed): *Surgical Dressings and Wound Healing*. London: Bradford University Press, 1971.

92. Haughey RE, Lammers RL, Wagner DK: Use of antibiotics in the initial management of soft tissue hand wounds. *Ann Emerg Med* 1981;10:187.

93. Hawkins J, Paris PM, Stewart RD: Mammalian bites. *Postgrad Med* 1983;73:52.

94. Heller MB: Management of bites: Dog, cat, human, and snake. *Resident Staff Physician* Feb 1982;75.

95. Herniman PD: Skin sensitisation by surgical adhesives. In Harkiss KJ (ed): *Surgical Dressings and Wound Healing*. London: Bradford University Press, 1981, pp 117–123.

96. Higham M: Infection in a puncture wound after it "Healed." *Hosp Pract* 1983;18:47.

97. Hildred SJ, Henderson CJ: Does antibiotic spray reduce wound infection? *Br Med J* 1977;53:122.

98. Hoffer ED: Tricks of the trade. *Emerg Med* 1984; 16(20):495.

99. Holm A, Zachariae L: Fingertip lesions, an evaluation of conservative treatment versus free skin grafting. *Acta Orthop Scand* 1974;45:382.

100. *Holy Bible, RSV—an Ecumenical Edition*. New York: Collins, 1973.

101. Houston AN, Roy WA, Faust RA, et al.: Tetanus prophylaxis in the treatment of puncture wounds of patients in the Deep South. *J Trauma* 1962;2:439.

102. Huang ET, Gilmore OJ, Reid C, et al.: Absence of bacterial resistance to povidone iodine. *J Clin Pathol* 1976; 29:752.

103. Hunt TK, Dunphy FE: *Fundamentals of Wound Management*. New York: Appleton-Century-Crofts, 1979.

104. Hunt TK, Van Winkle W: Normal repair. In Hunt TK, Dunphy JE (eds): *Fundamentals of Wound Management*. Norwalk, CT: Appleton-Century-Crofts, 1979.

105. Hunt TK, Burns. In Hunt TK, Dunphy JE (eds): *Fundamentals of Wound Management*. Norwalk, CT: Appleton-Century-Crofts, 1979.

106. Hunt TK: Disorders of repair and their management. In Hunt TK, Dunphy JE, (eds): *Fundamentals of Wound Management*. New York: Appleton-Century-Crofts, 1979.

107. Jacobs RF, Adelman L, Sack CM, et al.: Management of Pseudomonas osteochondritis complicating puncture wounds of the foot. *Pediatrics* 1982;69:432.

108. Jaffe AC: Animal bites. *Pediatr Clin North Am* 1983;30:405.

109. Jamra FN, Khuri S: The treatment of fingertip injuries. *J Trauma* 1970;11:749.

110. Jarvis WR, Banko S, Snyder E, et al.: *Pasteurella multocida* osteomyelitis following dog bites. *Am J Dis Child* 1981;135:625. July 1981.

111. Johanson PH: Pseudomonas infections of the foot following puncture wounds. *JAMA* 1968;204:170.

112A. Kaplan: *Emergency Management of Skin and Soft Tissue Wounds*. Little, Brown.

112B. Karlson TA: Incidence of facial injuries from dog bites. *JAMA* 1984;251:3265.

113. Keim D: Lecture on animal bites. 1981.

114. Kim Y: A new surgical technique. *Surg Gyn Obstet* 1973;137:669.

115. Koopman CF, Coulthard SW: Management of hematomas of the auricle. *Laryngoscope* 1979;89:1172.

116. L'Allemand D, Gruters A, Heidemann P, et al.: Iodine-induced alterations of thyroid function in newborn infants after prenatal and perinatal exposure to povidone iodine. *J Pediatr* 1983;102:935.

117. Lamon RP, Cicedro JJ, Frascone RJ, et al.: Open treatment of fingertip amputations. *Ann Emerg Med* 1983; 12:358.

118. Lang AG, Petterson HA: Osteomyelitis following puncture wounds of the foot in children. *J Trauma* 1976;16:993.

119. Larsen JS, Ulin AW: Tensile strength advantage of the far-and-near suture technique. *Surg Gyn Obstet* 1970;123.

120. Lauer EA, White WC, Lauer BA: Dog bites. *Am J Dis Child* 1982;136:202.

121. Lawrence JC: What materials for dressings? *Injury* 1982;13:500.

122. Leads from the MMWR: Rabies postexposure prophylaxis with human diploid cell rabies vaccine: Lower neutralizing antibody titers with Wyeth vaccine. *JAMA* 1985;253:1537.

123. Lerwick E: Studies on the efficacy and safety of polydioxanone monofilament absorbable suture. *Surg Gynecol Obstet* 1983;156:51.

124. Lindsey D, Nava C, Mari M: Effectiveness of penicillin irrigation in control of infection in sutured lacerations. *J Trauma* 1982;22:186.

125. Linsky CB, Rovee DT, Dow T: Effects of dressings on wound inflammation and scar tissue. In Dineen P, Hildick-Smith G (eds): *The Surgical Wound*. Philadelphia: Lea & Febiger, 1981.

126. Lividas DP, Piperingos GD, Sfontouris J, et al.: Lack of influence of povidone-iodine on tests of thyroid function. *J Intern Med Res* 1978;6:406.

127. Louis DS, Palmer AK, Burney RE: Open treatment of digital tip injuries. *JAMA* 1980;244:697.

128. Lynch MC, Dorgan JC: A case of *Pseudomonas aeruginosa* osteomyelitis of the tarsal cuboid following a penetrating wound of the foot in childhood. *Injury* 1983;14:354.

129. MacKinnon AE: Pseudomonas osteomyelitis following puncture wounds. *Postgrad Med* 1975;51:33.

130. Magee C, Rodeheaver GT, Edgerton MT, et al.: Studies of the mechanisms by which epinephrine damages tissue defenses. *J Surg Res* 1977;23:126.

131. Malinkowski: *J Trauma* 1979;19:655.

132. Mann RJ, Hoffeld TA, Farmer CB: Human bites of the hand: Twenty years of experience. *J Hand Surg* 1977; 2:97.

133. Marcy SM: Special series: Management of pediatric infectious diseases in office practice: Infections due to dog and cat bites. *Pediatr Infect Dis* 1982;1:351.

134. Margileth AM: Cat-scratch disease update. *AJDC* 1984;138:711.

135. Margileth AW, Wear DJ, Hadfield TL, et al.: Cat-scratch disease: Bacteria in skin at the primary inoculation site. *JAMA* 1984;252:928.

136. Meyer SW: *Functional Bandaging Including Splints and Protective Dressings*. New York: American Elsevier, 1967.

137. Morgan WJ: Povidone-iodine spray for wounds sutured in the accident department. *Lancet* 1969;1:769.

138. Mullikend JB, Healey NA, Glowacki J: Povidone-iodine and tensile strength of wounds in rats. *J Surg* 1980; 20:323.

139. Ordog GJ, Balasubramanium S, Wasserberger J: Rat bites: Fifty cases. *Ann Emerg Med* 1985;14:126.

140. Palmer J, Rees M: Dog bites of the face: A 15 year review. *Br J Plast Surg* 1983;36:315.

141. Peeples E, Boswick JA, Scott FA: Wounds of the hand contaminated by human or animal saliva. *J Trauma* 1980;20:383.

142. Peloso OS, Wilkinson LH: The chain stitch knot. *Surg Gynecol Obstet* 1974;139:599.

143. Peterson HS, Tressler HA, Lang AG, et al.: Fracture conference, puncture wounds of the foot. *Minn Med* 1973;56:787.

144. Polin K, Shulman ST: *Eikenella corrodens* osteomyelitis. *Pediatr* 1982;70:462.

145. Reed BR, Clark RAF: Cutaneous tissue repair: Practical implications of current knowledge. II. *J Am Acad Dermatol* 1985;13:919.

146. Rest JG, Goldstein EJC: Management of human animal bite wounds. *Emerg Med Clin North Am* 1985;3:117.

147. Riegler HF, Routson GW: Complications of deep puncture wounds of the foot. *J Trauma* 1979;19:18.

148. Roberts AHN, Teddy PJ: A prospective trial of prophylactic antibiotics in hand lacerations. *Br J Surg* 1977; 64:394.

149. Robson MC, Schmidt D, Heggers JP: Cefamandole therapy in hand infections. *J Hand Surg* 1983;8:560.

150. Rodeheaver GT, Halverson JM, Edlich RF: Mechanical performance of wound closure tapes. *Ann Emerg Med* 1983;12:203.

151. Rodeheaver GT, Kurtz L, Kircher BJ, et al.: Pluronic F-68: A promising new skin wound cleanser. *Ann Emerg Med* 1980;9:572.

152. Rodeheaver GT, Pettry D, Thacker JG, et al.: Wound cleansing by high pressure irrigation. *Surg Gynecol Obstet* 1975;141:357.

153. Rogers DM, Blouin GS, O'Leary JP: Povidone-iodine wound irrigation and wound sepsis. *Surg Gynecol Obstet* 1983;157:426.

154. Rosen P (ed): *Emergency Medicine: Concepts and Clinical Practice*. St. Louis: CV Mosby, 1983.

155. Rosen RA: The use of antibiotics in the initial management of recent dog-bite wounds. *Am J Emerg Med* 1985;3:19.

156. Safram M, Braverman LE: Effect of chronic douching with polyvinylpyrrolidone-iodine on iodine absorption and thyroid function. *Obstet Gynecol* 1982;60:35.

157. Sanford DD: Puncture wounds of the foot. *Am Fam Physician* 1981;24:119.

158. Scales JR: The clinical evaluation of adhesive dressings and plasters. In Harkiss KJ (ed): *Surgical Dressings and Wound Healing*. London: Bradford University Press, 1971, pp 102–116.

159. Scherr DD, Dodd TA: In vitro bacteriological evaluation of the effectiveness of antimicrobial irrigating solutions. *J Bone Joint Surg* 1975;120.

160. Schields D, Patzakis MJ, Meyers JH, et al.: Hand infections secondary to human bites. *J Trauma* 1975;15:235.

161. Schmidt DR, Heckman JD: *Eikenella corrodens* in human bite infections of the hand. *J Trauma* 1983;23:178.

162. Scott JE: Amputation of the finger. *Br J Surg* 1974; 61:574.

163. Seropian R, Reynolds B: Wound infection after preoperative depilatory versus razor preparation. *Am J Surg* 1971;121:251.

164. Sharp VW, Belden TA, King PH, et al.: Suture resistance to infection. *Surgery* 1982;91:61.

165. Siebert WT, Dewan S, Williams TW: Case report Pseudomonas puncture wound osteomyelitis in adults. *Am J Med Sci* 1982;238:83.

166. Simon RR, Brenner BE: *Procedures and Techniques in Emergency Medicine*. Baltimore: Williams & Wilkins, 1982.

167. Simpson BJ, Winter GD: A method of studying the performance of dressings using a standard wound in the domestic pig. In *Surgical Dressings and Wound Healing*. Harkiss KJ (ed.): London: Bradford University Press, 1971, pp 70–77.

168. Sindelar WF, Mason GR: Efficacy of povidone-iodine irrigation in prevention of surgical wound infections. *Surg Forum* 1977;28:48.

169. Sindelar WF, Mason GR: Irrigation of subcutaneous tissue with povidone-iodine solution for prevention of surgical wound infections. *Surg Gynecol Obstet* 1979;148:227.

170. Spira M, Hardy SB: Management of the injured ear. *Am J Surg* 1963;106:678.

171. State of California Department of Health Records: *Cases of Animal Rabies by County and Species, January 1, 1984–December 31, 1984*. Infectious Disease Section, California Department of Health Services.

172. Stegman SJ: Fifteen ways to close surgical wounds. *J Dermatol Surg* 1975;1:25.

173. Stevenson TR, Thacker JG, Rodeheaver GT, et al.: Cleansing the traumatic wound by high pressure syringe irrigation. *JACEP* 1976;5:17.

174. Strassburg MA, Greenland S, Marron JA, et al.: Animal bites: Patterns of treatment. *Ann Emerg Med* 1981; 10:193.

175. Strauch B, Sharzer LA, Petro J, et al.: Replantation of Amputated Parts of the Penis, Nose, Ear, and Scalp. *Clin Plast Surg* 1983;10:115.

176. Swanson NA, Tromovitch TA: Suture materials, 1980: Properties, uses, and abuse. *Int J Dermatol* 1982; 21:373.

177. Tandberg D: Glass in the hand and foot, will an x-ray film show it? *JAMA* 1982;248:1872.

178. Taylor GA: Management of human bite injuries of the hand. *Can Med Assoc J* 1985;133:191.

179. Thomson HG, Svitek V: Small animal bites: The role of primary closure. *J Trauma* 1972;13:20.

180. Thorndike A: *A Manual of Bandaging, Strapping and Splinting*, ed 3. Philadelphia: Lea & Febiger, 1959.

181. Tindall JP, Harrison CM: *Pasteurella multocida* infections following animal injuries, especially cat bites. *Arch Dermatol* 1972;105:412.

182. Tobin GR: Closure of contaminated wounds—biologic and technical considerations. *Surg Clin North Am* 1984;64:639.

183. Trevaskis AE, Rempei J, Okunski W, et al.: Sliding subcutaneous-pedicle flaps to close a circular defect. *Plast Reconstr Surg* 1970;46:155.

184. Veitch JM, Omer GE: Case report: Treatment of cat-bite injuries of the hand. *J Trauma* 1979;19:201.

185. Viljanto J: Disinfection of surgical wounds without inhibition of normal wound healing. *Arch Surg* 1980; 115:253.

186. Wayne MA: Clinical evaluation of Epi-Lock—a semiocclusive dressing. *Ann Emerg Med* 1985;14:20.

187. Weston WJ: Thorn and twig-induced pseudotumors of bone and soft tissues. *Br J Radiol* 1963;36:323.

188. Wheeler CB, Rodeheaver GT, Thacker JG: Side-effects of high-pressure irrigation. *Surg Gynecol Obstet* 1976;143:775.

189. White WB, Iserson KV, Criss E: Topical anesthesia for laceration repair: Tetracaine versus TAC (tetracaine, adrenaline, and cocaine). *Am J Emerg Med* 1986;4:319.

190. Winter GD: Healing of skin wounds and the influence of dressings on the repair process. In Harkiss KJ (ed.): *Surgical Dressings and Wound Healing.* London: Bradford University Press, 1971, pp 46–60.

191. Worlock P, Boland P, Darrell J, et al.: The role of prophylactic antibiotics following hand injuries. *Br J Clin Pract* 1980;34:290.

192. Zacher JB: Management of injuries of the distal phalanx. *Surg Clin North Am* 1984;64:747.

193. Zamora JL: Povidone-iodine and wound infection, editorial. *Surgery* 1984;95:121.

194. Zook EG, Miller M, Ban Beek AL, et al.: Successful treatment protocol for canine fang injuries. *J Trauma* 1980;20.

195. Rosen P: personal communication.

196. Gravett A, Sterner S, Clinton JE, et al.: A trial of povidone-iodine in the prevention of infection in sutured lacerations. *Ann Emerg Med* 1987;16:167.

197. Gilman AG, Goodman LS, Rall TW, et al.: *Goodman and Gilman's The Pharmacological Basis of Therapeutics*, 7th ed, New York: Macmillan, 1985.

Index

153